Hand Maintenance Guide

for Massage Therapists

Shogo Mochizuki

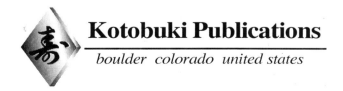

Kotobuki Publications

boulder colorado united states

Hand Maintenance Guide
for Massage Therapists

Published in the United States by

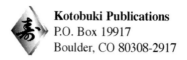 **Kotobuki Publications**
P.O. Box 19917
Boulder, CO 80308-2917

ISBN : 1-57615-075-5
Library of Congress Cataloging-in-Publication Data

NOTE TO THE READER:

All materials and instructions contained in this book require supervised training by a qualified professional. The authors, publisher or Japanese Massage & Bodywork Institute are not responsible for the effects of the procedures contained in this book. All matters regarding your health require medical supervision; these materials are not a substitute for qualified care or treatment.

Printed in United States of America

First Edition

3 5 7 6 4 2

Hand Maintenance Guide for Massage Therapists, version 1.2

An Ounce of Prevention
is Worth a Pound of Cure

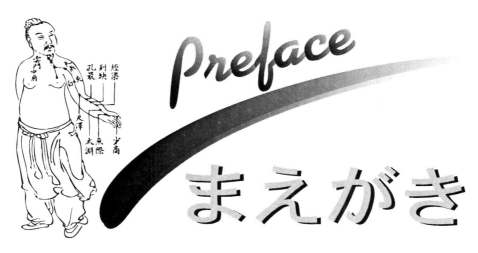

Preface

まえがき

While teaching in the United States, I have seen many skillful massage practitioners and students leave the field because of problems with the wrists, hands, or fingers. Several of these problems could have been prevented if they had applied simple hand maintenance and massage techniques. Many practitioners spend enormous amounts of time, energy, and money on training and education, but few realize the importance of taking precautions to maintain the health of their hands.

I want to explain here the kinds of movements that should be avoided because they can lead to problems in the wrists, hands, and fingers. I also want to present a series of techniques that help avoid difficulties for people who use their hands all the time. Daily practice of this simple routine should prevent, reduce, and possibly eliminate hand problems for the therapist.

This book was originally developed to aid my anma and other Japanese bodywork classes due to the very intense hand manipulations required for massage techniques. This information can be particularly valuable for professional practitioners, regardless of the style of massage they use. Additionally, these techniques help eliminate potential problems as beginning students start to use their hands and fingers more extensively and build the hand-muscle strength—it is very important to learn safe and proper techniques from the beginning. This book contains anatomical terminology. If you are a beginning student or a layperson, please refer to an anatomy textbook for an explanation of these terms.

The first step in massage education is learning hand maintenance. It is an important lesson in every class I teach, no matter what style of bodywork I am presenting. I am surprised at how many people—people who have recently graduated from massage school or even therapists who have been practicing for years—lack this knowledge. It is my hope that these techniques benefit students, massage therapists, health care professionals, and others outside the classroom.

Shogo Mochizuki
Spring 1999

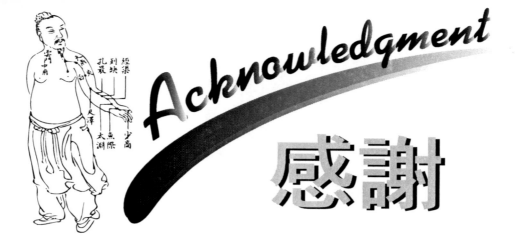

Acknowledgment

感謝

I have many people to thank for their help in the process of creating this book, This book would not have been possible without each person's unique contribution.

I would like to thank my grandmother for sharing her knowledge and guidance with me and for leading me to the study and practice of traditional Japanese medicine and massage. I thank my family members and ancestors who have practiced traditional medicine for more than two centuries. Also, thank you to my parents for their support over the years.

Thank you to all my masters who taught me knowledge and wisdom from a different perspective beyond my original understanding of massage technique.

Special thanks to Jeffrey Stevens, senior editor of Kotobuki Publications. Also, a very special thank you to Deborahann Smith for her outstanding work editing this book. Thank you to Kevin McGowan for doing a wonderful job with the technical editing.

Thank you to Andrew Borsick, Gregory Hill, and others for proofing this book.

Thank you to Shinji Tsuji for his wonderful photographic contributions.

Thanks to all my friends who have helped me in numerous ways and to the many people who have supported my practice over the years. Also, my deepest appreciation goes out to all the staff and students of the various massage schools who have supported our ongoing education and have made our workshops possible.

And I would like to thank you, the reader, for your support.

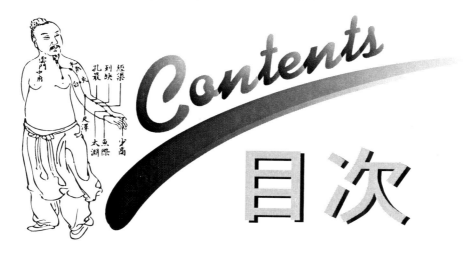

Contents

目次

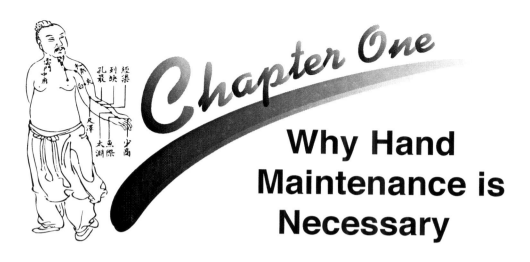

Chapter One

Why Hand Maintenance is Necessary

In 713 A.D., the Japanese government established the first massage school in Japan, based on 1,000 years of massage techniques and education passed on from the Chinese. In the last 1,300 years, Japanese massage schools have built upon this foundation, developing effective massage education.

An elementary lesson in any Japanese massage school includes how to maintain optimal health for your hands. Although each instructor may have a slightly different method, these basic techniques have been passed on for centuries and are essential for a long and successful career as a massage therapist.

When I began teaching Japanese massage and bodywork, students often asked, "What can I do for the pain in my hands?" or "When I give more than two massages a day, I have stiff forearms or painful wrists the next day. What can I do to help this?"

If I asked them, 'Do you warm up your hands and forearms prior to giving massage?' usually the answer would be "no" or "I didn't know I needed to warm up my hands." I told them that warming up was essential for maintaining the hands. You can't just show up at your office five minutes prior to your client's arrival, put sheets on a table, and go to work. You are doing four to six hours of massage with the hands, arms, and shoulders and they must be warmed up before doing the work. Then I inquired, 'Do you warm your hands after the massage?' Again, the answer was "no." When I ask, 'so what do you do to maintain your hands?' The response was usually, "Nothing, how do you do that?"

Generally, massage schools in the United States do not teach the basics of hand maintenance as they do in Japan. It is no surprise that many Western practitioners develop aches and pains during training, because they aren't taught how to avoid these problems. I believe that any form of oil-based Western massage is even harder on the practitioner's hands than the no-oil Eastern massage; oil-based massage requires repetitive pushing, whereas Eastern massage relies more on pulling techniques.

In Japan, massage students become therapists after graduation and continue to work in this capacity for the rest of their lives. In the United States, however, therapists rarely practice for more than ten years. Why? Because massage schools don't teach appropriate techniques for maintaining the therapists' health. One survey shows that more than seventy percent of American practitioners leave the field within seven years of graduation, **with hand or wrist problems being the number one cause.**

The problem stems in part from the fact that many massage schools in the United States have been established for only a few decades; they have not yet developed teaching methods of their own, nor do they have the accumulated experience or information that is available to Asian therapists. Also, many Western instructors have only been practicing and teaching massage for a few years, and they lack the solid knowledge and experience required to adequately teach. However, many of the massage schools in Japan are several hundred years old and the massage instructors have been teaching massage for thirty or forty years or longer. Likewise, the students usually begin their studies very early. For instance, I began learning massage at the age of four and have practiced massage ever since. During this time, I have developed my hand and arm strength and practiced techniques for self-maintenance, so I can work on more than fifty clients a week without experiencing pain or difficulties with my hands.

If you work as a professional massage therapist and spend years building your business and clientele, you can't afford to have hand problems that jeopardize your practice. Basically, your business is dependent on your hands. Obviously, one of the most important reasons for hand maintenance is the protection of your career. If you rely on your hands for your occupation, you need to take care of them as if they were your most precious possessions. For massage therapists, the hands are the primary "tools of the trade," just as an auto mechanic works every day with his or her tools. Eventually the auto mechanic's wrenches and screwdrivers wear out, at which point the mechanic replaces them with new ones and business continues as usual. However, the tools—hands, wrists, and forearms—of massage therapists must not wear out because they cannot be replaced.

Any traditional art in Japan must be learned in the steps and stages of discipline. Each step has deep meaning which developed over centuries of teaching experience. For example, when you practice judo, you first learn to protect yourself because if you don't properly master defense techniques, you will get injured. The same is true with the art of massage—first you must master self-protection and maintenance to prevent injury to yourself. An important philosophy of Japanese massage is that there are many opportunities to express the freedom and quality of your art. But you must master all basics beginning with self-protection. **No techniques are worth performing if they are harmful to your hands, regardless of the benefit to your client.**

If you work as a full-time professional massage therapist, it often means treating twenty to thirty clients per week or more. This means three to five clients and four to six hours of massage each day, much of which requires hard work for the arms, wrists, and hands. If the forearms get this much regular exercise, it is important to keep them loose and flexible by thoroughly warming them up prior to the massage. This is like professional athletes who spend large amounts of time warming up, stretching, and getting loose before they work out and before they perform. A marathon runner does not start running without preparation; he or she thoroughly trains and stretches the legs before the race.

Human hands can endure decades upon decades of hard labor if they are treated properly. But if hands are put through repetitive motions and continual stress without proper maintenance, they will not last a decade; in fact, they may be ready to retire in two or three years. Often students say if they develop hand problems or carpal tunnel syndrome they will have the problem corrected through surgery. I am not convinced that this "quick fix" is the answer. In fact, when hands are injured from overwork, it is unlikely that they will heal to a condition where they can be used again for full-time massage work, regardless of surgery. It is better to learn hand maintenance basics. For your health, your happiness, and your career, please take good care of your hands!

I have been practicing acupuncture and Japanese massage for many years, and I have come across countless examples of over-stressed forearms, wrists, and hands. I have done what I could to reverse these conditions, but the sad fact of the matter is that injuries to these areas are not easy to treat—it is easier to prevent hand problems than it is to fix these problems once they have begun. Wrist problems are especially difficult to repair and cure. When a problem does arise, it can be treated so that it does not inhibit the regular activities of daily life, such as opening jars or writing with a pencil, but to resume a full-time or even part-time massage practice in the face of these problems often requires extensive treatment and time for recuperation.

When someone is fortunate enough to receive the care necessary for proper healing or if the condition improves on its own, it is still likely that the condition will recur. Why? Because the techniques and routines that provoked the affliction are usually those that the therapist has grown accustomed to—and those on which the massage sessions depend—so the therapist naturally returns to these techniques. Therefore, in order to avoid a condition's recurrence, it is important to develop a hand maintenance routine comprised of a warm-up period prior to the massage and a post-session period of specific stretches and self-massage techniques.

Hand maintenance generally consists of two areas: 1) constantly correcting body and hand positions to prevent problems, which I explain in Chapter Two and; 2) employing a series of massaging and stretching exercises for the hands, fingers, wrists, forearms, upper arms, shoulders, and neck as a way to keep the therapist in optimum condition. These routines vary, depending on individual needs. In Chapter Three, I demonstrate an example of a routine that is general enough to work for the majority of people.

Hand maintenance routines aren't used only to prevent problems, but are intended to warm up the hand, wrist, and forearm in preparation for giving the massage. Many therapists feel that after half an hour or an hour into giving massage the hands and arms loosen up. This means that, during the warm-up time, they are not giving a quality massage. For example, in traditional Japanese medicine, ki (human energy) flows with blood. Tight muscles decrease blood flow, so the energy does not flow as well to the hand. Warming up the hands is important for effective treatment, regardless of whether there are hand problems or not.

If you feel somewhat stiff in the forearms in the morning, it is absolutely essential that you do not attempt massage work until you have softened and stretched the connective tissues of your forearms, wrists, and hands. Do not tell yourself that these muscles will warm up on their own as you go about your morning tasks; this may be somewhat true for general use of the arms, but intensive use of the arms, as in massage therapy, requires the muscles to be thoroughly warmed up prior to giving a massage.

It is unwise to place stress on a cold, tight muscle because when a muscle is tight, it does not extend or flex properly; if it is pressured to do so, it may tear. Tears in the muscular fibers can cause soreness, pain, or restriction of movement. Although this affliction does not necessarily damage tissue permanently, it can cause intense pain and virtually rule out any possibility of continuing massage work. So remember, **take care of your hands!**

Chapter Two

The Causes of Problems

I teach the traditional Japanese massage styles of anma and shiatsu. These traditions are based on a foundation of training that allows for creativity and freedom. To manifest this creativity and freedom, the practitioner must respect the basic limitations of his or her body's capacity to give massage. Once you understand the foundation and your limits, you can improvise with your clients however you like, giving them a very special treatment without risk of harming your body or the client.

A person may have difficulties giving massage for several reasons. It is normal for professional therapists to feel occasional pain in the hands and arms; however, if a therapist experiences constant pain, it is a signal that difficulties are caused by previous injuries, insufficient development of musculature (through training and practice), genetic weaknesses in hands and arms, overuse of the muscles with lack of proper hand maintenance, or improper use of hands and arms during massage.

Sometimes a therapist may encounter pain that can be traced back to a particular injury suffered in that part of the body. In this case, it is best to modify whatever massage techniques exacerbate the problem or avoid them altogether. However, if it is possible to rehabilitate an injury, by all means, take the steps to do so. The hand maintenance exercises in this book are helpful, but you may want to consider acupuncture or other treatments as well.

While it is true that in Asia many professional therapists can handle forty or more client sessions per week, it is only because they have been thoroughly trained over a period of years. Just as a pianist who has been practicing piano from early childhood has extraordinary hand strength compared to someone who took up piano as an adult, massage therapists cannot expect to quickly force the development of the hand, arm, shoulder, and back strength. It takes many years of careful practice to do deep massage work without risking personal injury. If your body is only able to give two quality massages a day, don't attempt more and remember that your body will accumulate strength over time. Forcing more massage work than you can comfortably handle not only results in an ineffective massage but may cause physical damage to your body.

If you examine the hands of ten different people, you will notice that every person has a different physiological development. Although the anatomy is basically the same, the expression of it is unique to each individual. For example, some people have delicate bone development, while others have sturdy bone development. Also, some people have strong bone development but weak bone alignment. In other words, there are certain physiological conditions that are conducive to being a massage therapist, and there are certain conditions that make it difficult to do massage work without encountering pain and injury. Once again, this is an individual matter. There are small people who are able to deliver endless sessions of deep massage without the slightest trouble and there are big, strong people who cannot handle more than a session every few days.

Pain in the fingers and hands is an indicator that you have applied more pressure than your body is able to manage. As my Japanese teachers continually emphasized, it is very important to learn to **listen to your hands!** Your body will send messages of overstress or improper use of strength well before a serious injury develops. If you pay attention to these signals as they appear, a painful condition can usually be avoided by a change in the alignment of your fingers, hands, and bones or through a modification of technique or correcting a tendency to hyperextend a joint. These adjustments can be applied during a session immediately as they arise. Pay attention to the signals your body sends you; do not continue with a technique if it causes pain. Your body is trying to engage you in a cooperative dialogue so that it can deliver the best possible massage without harm.

It is also important to appreciate your limitations and not take on more than you can physically handle. For example, if you are able to handle only three sessions a day, do not schedule four. If you begin to develop stress or pain in your hands or arms or if you feel that a part of your body is unusually fatigued, allow yourself to take time off from performing massage. Please do not avoid resting from massage when it feels necessary. If you try to "work through" the pain, you may have to leave massage altogether when injuries develop.

Massage relies on the strength of the rotator cuff muscles of the back and shoulders. These muscles are built for heavier work over an extended period of time than hands, wrists, or forearms. If, after a day of massage sessions, you feel sore or tight in this area, it is a normal indicator you are relying on these muscles for the strength that massage requires. If, however, your soreness or tightness is primarily in your hands, wrists, and forearms, it indicates you are providing strength from the weaker muscles of your arm; this will definitely cause problems sooner or later. It is essential to understand proper body mechanics if you intend to grow as a practitioner.

In Japan, one of the first massage lessons involves correct body positioning and mechanics for hand manipulation techniques. Protecting the body and hands is always of primary concern when giving a massage. It is important to study with an instructor who has a genuine understanding of body mechanics and can help you instill good postural habits from the beginning. Therefore, I do not recommend self-taught massage at the beginning level. Rather, you should meet with an experienced teacher to analyze your own body mechanics and learn to give massage from the appropriate muscle groups; this will allow the massage techniques to have the deepest effect and it helps your body to grow stronger and more relaxed over the years of practice. Once you have acquired good habits, they will stay with you. But if you begin with bad habits, they are very difficult to change.

Learning the proper positioning and movements in the beginning of your massage education is vital for building a solid foundation of good habits. You must also learn to avoid bad habits—such as applying techniques from an improper position—because improperly applied techniques can strain or damage a therapist's soft tissue and cause premature wear on the joints.

If your body positioning is correct, you can use your body weight more comfortably to give a smoother massage. But if your body mechanics are wrong, you push with your upper body and arms to accomplish a movement that can only be delivered smoothly when the entire body is coordinated. If you become overly fatigued during or after a session, it indicates you are using your body inefficiently and you need to readjust your body mechanics. To avoid forming bad habits, it is advisable to install mirrors in your massage room so you can analyze your body mechanics from time to time.

When you maintain proper body mechanics, your body can coordinate itself to movements through overall relaxation. The best body mechanics involve using a minimum amount of effort. Master therapists can apply a technique with incredible subtlety and effectiveness because their bodies are deeply relaxed and completely coordinated, working as a unit. However, beginning therapists tend to have more rigid movements and sometimes work with a "jerky" quality; this is a result of incomplete relaxation, which causes a lack of coordination. Rigid, tense muscles pull joints together, causing compression in the areas that need to be most fluid. The body works against itself when joints are compressed, pulling in other muscles for movement, whereas relaxation provides a fluidity to the joints and calls on only the muscles that are optimal for delivering an effective massage. Because working in this way is actually restful to the body, the practitioner can handle more work. Remember, proper body mechanics are designed to let the body relax, which in turn allows the natural strength of the body to emerge through the coordination of various muscle groups.

It is very important to avoid hand, wrist, elbow, or shoulder injuries, especially if you support yourself and your family with your massage profession. It is also best to avoid any activities that can easily cause hand or elbow injuries. Furthermore, it is essential to take time off to rest properly and also to receive proper treatment if you have injured your wrist, elbow, or shoulders. If you continue to work when you have an injury or pain, it can result in more severe and long-term problems.

Contraindicated Movement in Massage Therapy

Although individual Japanese instructors and massage schools emphasize different hand and arm techniques for massage, there are agreed-upon advisories of what therapists should avoid so as not to injury themselves. Several contraindicated hand movements are known to cause injury; but there are thirteen general contraindicated movements which are most visible in present-day massage therapy among practitioners in the West.

The most common problems therapists encounter are those of the thumbs and wrists. The first four of these contraindicated examples represent common mistakes that lead to thumb injuries. In my own experience, I have found that it is better to use finger applications instead of thumb applications wherever possible, with the exception of straight downward-pressure applications. In my own therapy, I have gradually learned to work out applications which substitute finger and palm techniques for thumb techniques. Nowadays, I am able to employ finger manipulation for many applications that have been known to cause strain when applied with the thumbs. If you use your thumbs for certain techniques, there is one piece of advice that I want to emphasize: as soon as you begin to feel fatigue in the thenar muscle (the pad beneath the thumb) **stop immediately**, and do not use the thumb again until the pain has subsided completely.

The next six examples address the ways in which therapists commonly jeopardize their wrists. The wrist is a fragile joint which, in contrast to the elbow, shoulders, or knee, does not have major muscle support. In my experience, the wrist seems to be the most problematic joint for many therapists.

It is important to pay attention to the various forms of tension we inflict on our joints during a session. For example, when you press against a client's muscle, you cause some degree of compression in your wrist joint. Although this is not possible or necessary to avoid altogether, there are many times when, instead of pushing against a muscle, the therapist can come from the opposite side of the muscle and pull against it. This creates space in your own wrist joint, rather than generating compression. This is not just true of the wrists, but of the joints of the fingers, elbows, and shoulders. If you can find a way to pull against a client's muscle rather than push against it, you reduce the compression in the joints involved.

If you apply very light pressure with any application, it is not likely to cause problems. But once you apply heavier pressure, there will be heavier pressure between your joints, which makes you more susceptible to injury. As you increase pressure, your hand and wrist should be stabilized to support the fingers properly, adjusting the angle of the fingers against the surface to avoid undue pressure to the finger pad. By slightly overlapping your fingers, you can give them better support and avoid hyperextensions that can cause injuries.

The following explanations highlight what you should avoid. Ultimately you want to integrate these guidelines into your technique so you don't need to think about them while performing massage. Until then, apply yourself to practicing the guidelines—even if it seems tedious at first, it will make you a more capable therapist. Remember, it takes quite a while for some bad habits to give rise to symptoms and injury. Don't continue with bad habits just because they haven't caused harm yet: **they soon will, and by doing so will also detract from the massage.**

1. Do not rotate the thumb from the carpometacarpal or metacarpophalangeal joint

Improper Technique
Applying pressure with the thumb and then rotating the thumb from the carpometacarpal or the metacarpophalangeal joints.

When the thumb moves by itself with extremely light pressure, it is not as much of a problem. However, deeper pressure can cause strain.

Problem
Rotation while applying pressure causes the premature wear of the carpometacarpal and metacarpophalangeal joints by grinding away the cartilage between the bones; this can lead to bone directly contacting bone, which is very painful.

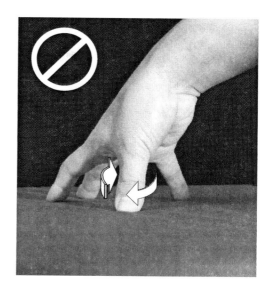

Proper Technique
Apply pressure with the thumb and then apply rotation with the thumb safely, the therapist must keep the entire hand in a fixed position and then **rotate the entire hand from either the elbow or shoulder joint.** Generally, the fingers of the same hand act as pivots for the entire hand or can be positioned to support the thumb during the rotation.

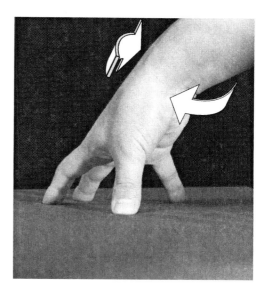

2. Do not apply pressure with a flexed thumb

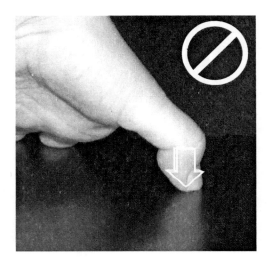

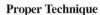

Some Western massage instructors and reflexologists seem to feel that this is an appropriate technique, it is definitely contraindicated in the Japanese massage tradition.

Improper Technique
Applying pressure with a flexed thumb.

Problem
Applying pressure with a flexed thumb causes an undue amount of stress to the interphalangeal, carpometacarpal, and metacarpophalangeal joints, as well as an undue amount of strain on the adductor pollicis, flexor pollicis brevis, opponens pollicis, and abductor pollicis brevis muscles. This improper technique can also lead to nerve compression in the interphalangeal joint of the thumb. Also, this position can bring the thumbnail into contact with the client's body.

Proper Technique
To safely apply pressure with the thumb, the therapist must keep the thumb in a straight, fixed position. Generally, the elbow should be positioned directly over the thumb when applying pressure to keep the joints of the thumb, hand, and wrist in a straight line and to minimize the amount of stress and strain to the joints and soft tissue.

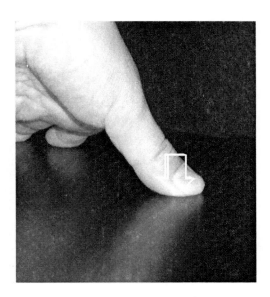

3. Do not apply pressure over the interphalangeal joint of the thumb

Some people are naturally able to hyperextend the interphalangeal joint of the thumb and may attempt to apply pressure with this joint. This can be very harmful to the therapist's hand.

Improper Technique
Applying pressure with or over the interphalangeal joint of the thumb.

Problem
Applying pressure over the interphalangeal joint of the thumb causes the interphalangeal, carpometacarpal, and metacarpophalangeal joints of the thumb to hyperextend, creating an undue amount of strain on the joints. This improper technique can also cause nerve compression in the interphalangeal joint of the thumb.

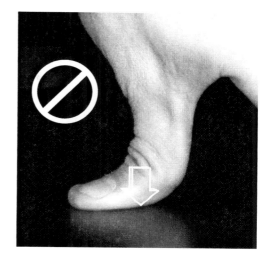

Proper Technique
To safely apply pressure with the thumb, the therapist should apply only light pressure with the pad and heavier pressure with the fingertip of the thumb, while keeping the thumb in a straight and fixed position. People who are able to hyperextend the interphalangeal joint of the thumbs very easily should keep the thumbs slightly flexed when applying pressure, and they should raise the palms of the hands off the client's body by finding a position for the supporting four fingers. Another way is to make a loose fist behind the thumb so that the interphalangeal joint is directly supported by the fingers. Generally, the elbow should be positioned directly over the thumb when applying pressure with the thumb, to keep the joints of the thumb, hand, and wrist in a straight line and to minimize the amount of stress and strain to the joints and soft tissue.

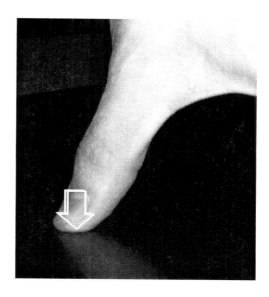

4. Do not hyperabduct the thumb

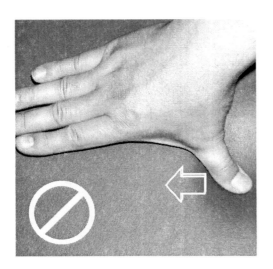

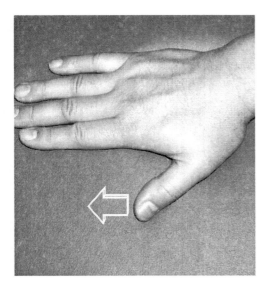

Improper Technique
Applying pressure or attempting to perform stroking techniques with an improperly supported thumb or with an improper part of the thumb, causing the thumb to be hyperabducted.

Problem
This can overstretch the adductor pollicis muscle, causing a strain or possible tear of the tendons and cartilage. The carpometacarpal joint of the thumb can also be unduly stressed and hypercompressed by the hyperabduction of the thumb.

Proper Technique
To safely apply pressure with the thumb or to use the thumb for stroking techniques, the therapist should only apply light pressure with the pad and heavier pressure with the thumb tip. It is important to keep the thumb in a straight and fixed position and the joints of the thumb, hand, and wrist in a straight line. Keeping the hand in a fixed position minimizes the amount of stress and strain to the joints and soft tissue. Keeping the joints in alignment helps the therapist to apply pressure in a properly supported manner.

5. Do not hyperextend the wrist

This problem is very common among massage thera-pists, and **wrist injuries are the number one reason for the premature end of a career as a massage therapist.** You must always avoid even momentary hyperextensions of the wrist, even when your not giving a massage.

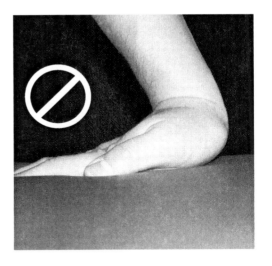

Improper Technique
Applying any technique with a hyperextended wrist.

Problem
Applying any technique with a hyperextended wrist can quickly cause severe problems for the therapist, in the muscles, ligaments, tendons, and fascia of the wrist, as well as the wrist joint itself. These problems can quickly spread to the hand and forearm, as the therapist tries to compensate for the injury to the wrist.

Proper Technique
The therapist should consciously minimize the angle of the wrist when applying any technique and keep the wrist as soft and flexible as possible. The therapist should not allow the angle between the back of the hand and the forearm to go below 90 degrees. The hand and body position should be adjusted throughout a massage to maintain a safe wrist angle and proper body mechanics. Simple adjustments during the massage can mean the difference between a lifelong career in massage or the premature end of a career as a massage therapist.

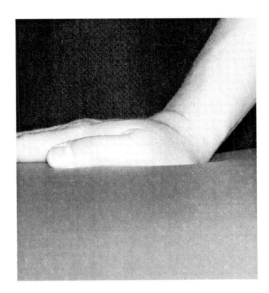

6. Do not hyperabduct or hyperadduct the wrist

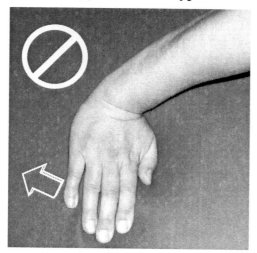

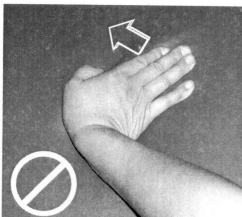

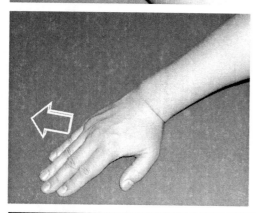

Hyperabduction and hyperadduction of the wrist can become more of a problem for practitioners of oil-based massage, especially during some effleurage techniques. For example, practitioners of Swedish massage are more prone to experience these problems than people who use massage techniques that do not use oil, such as anma or shiatsu.

Improper Technique

The hyperabduction and hyperadduction of the wrist when applying any technique.

Problem

Applying any technique with a hyperabducted or hyperadducted wrist can cause compression between the bones of the radius and ulna and the carpal bones they contact. Eventually this leads to painful nerve compression in the wrist. These improper positions compromise the alignment of the elbow and shoulder joints, which can also develop problems.

Proper Technique

The therapist should always try to minimize the angle of the wrist when applying any technique. It is important not to let the hand drag during long strokes because this can cause the wrist to hyperadduct or hyperabduct. Rather, keep a fixed wrist position (although not rigid), and stay within a safe range of motion throughout the stroke. If possible, when stroking, it is best to keep stroking in toward your body rather than away from you. The movement in stroking techniques should come from the shoulders and elbows and the coordinated movement of the entire body. This prevents the tendency to extend the arm through a stroke which can cause the wrist to go into unsafe abductions and adductions. The therapist must constantly adjust hand and body positions during a massage to maintain a safe wrist angle and proper body mechanics.

7. Do not support weight with the fingers when they are in a flexed position

This problem arises in conjunction with work on the base of the skull when the therapist is attempting to support the weight of the client's head and neck with flexed fingers. This also occurs during techniques that use the same hand position to drag in a superior direction against the erectors (client in supine position, therapist's hands between table and client's back) using the fingertips.

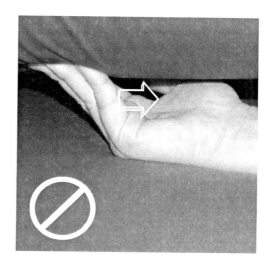

Improper Technique
Any technique that causes the joints of the fingers and hand to be compressed while in a flexed position.

Problem
The metacarpophalangeal joint is extremely vulnerable to injury while in this position, because the heads of the bones are in very close contact and cannot easily support weight without becoming hypercompressed.

Proper Technique
Hand position must be adjusted, with the palm turned inward to apply pressure with the lateral edge of the index finger and the index finger supported by the other three fingers, instead of applying pressure with the fingertips of the four fingers. If this is not possible, avoid the technique altogether rather than risking injury.

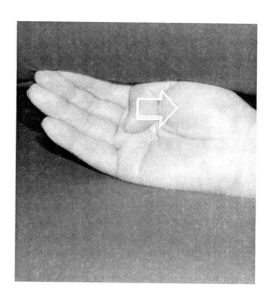

8. Do not apply any technique with the heel of your hand while the fingers and wrist are stiff

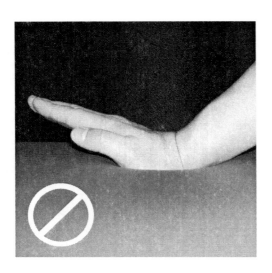

Improper Technique
Any application of pressure with the heel of the hand while your fingers and wrist are stiff.

Problem
Applying pressure with the heel of the hand while your fingers and wrist are stiff causes undue stress to the ligaments and tendons of the wrist.

Proper Technique
The wrist must be soft and flexible when applying pressure with the heel of the hand. The fingers should be relaxed and conform naturally to the contours of the client's body, minimizing stress to the tendons of the extensor muscles. Try to relax the elbow and shoulder joints and apply pressure using your body weight.

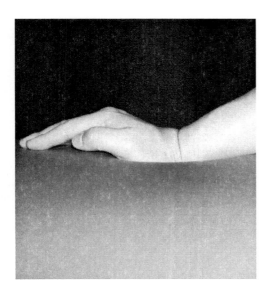

9. Do not apply pressure with the fist where the wrist could suddenly collapse

Improper Technique

Any technique that uses the fist while the wrist is unsupported with any hint of flexion in the wrist, or on an area that is unstable (such as the erector muscles, which can suddenly contract and throw the wrist into flexion or extension).

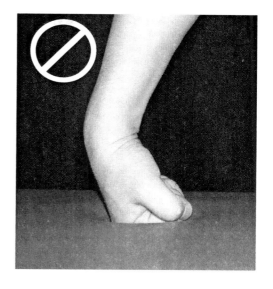

Problem

This can be dangerous to the therapist and the client, because the wrist may buckle in a number a different directions, causing serious damage to the muscles, ligaments, tendons, and fascia of the wrist, as well as the wrist joint itself. The wrist is extremely vulnerable to injury while in this position because it is not properly supported. The client is also at risk to injury because the therapist does not have sufficient control of the hand in this position and there is a large chance that the hand could slip while the wrist is unsupported.

Proper Technique

The therapist should grasp the wrist with the hand that is not applying the technique to provide the wrist with the necessary support and stabilization. If you have to use both fists on an area (although this is not recommended) be very careful to find the proper body position that allows the most stability. Otherwise, avoid the technique entirely.

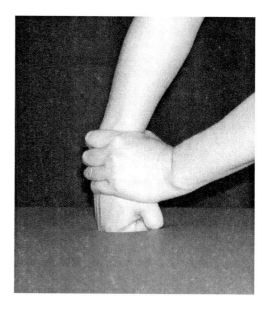

10. Do not rely on the wrist for movement and do not overuse the range of motion of the wrist

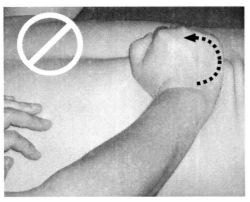

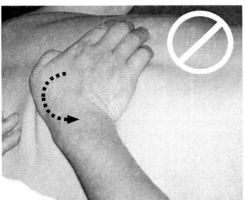

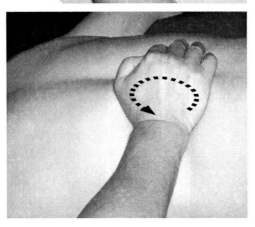

This can become a problem particularly for practitioners of anma and *tui-na* during rotation techniques, although Swedish massage practitioners can encounter this as well.

Improper Technique
In general, too much movement of the wrist during any technique, especially when the main movement should originate from the back, shoulder, and elbow joints.

Problem
Over-reliance on the wrist during therapy can cause a rapid movement between hyperadduction or hyperabduction of the wrist joints. This can cause compression between the bones of the radius and ulna and the carpal bones they contact.

Proper Technique
Minimize the movement of the wrist by relying more on the movement of the elbow and shoulders. Do not use the full range of motion of the wrist during massage; it is best to keep within a limited range so that the wrist is not jeopardized.

11. Do not hyperextend the fingers

Improper Technique

Applying pressure with improperly supported fingers, causing the fingers to hyperextend.

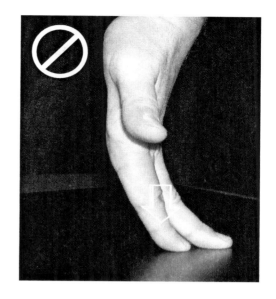

Problem

Applying pressure with improperly supported fingers, causing the fingers to hyperextend, can overstretch the tissue of the palm, creating strain or possible tears of the muscle fibers. The hyperextension of the fingers can also cause an undue amount of strain on the distal interphalangeal, proximal interphalangeal, and metacarpophalangeal joints. Insufficient hand strength may be a contributing factor to this problem.

Proper Technique

To safely apply pressure with the fingers, the therapist should support the fingers properly. An example of a way to support the fingers is to slightly overlap the fingers and then apply the pressure, so each finger supports the others. Another way is to slightly flex your fingers and hand when applying pressure or to use the outer edges of the index and middle fingers by rotating the wrist. These surfaces can support more pressure than the flexed fingers can.

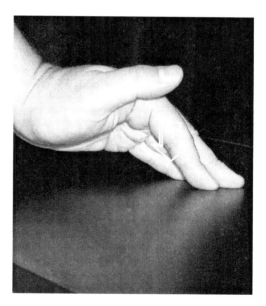

12. Do not repeat any one technique for too long a period of time in a session

Improper Technique

Overuse of a single technique during a single session.

Problem

Any single technique using a particular group of muscles will cause fatigue if that area is overtaxed by too much work. Using a single technique too much during a session does not allow these muscles to rest sufficiently and eventually leads to injury.

Proper Technique

Alternate different techniques when working the same area in order to bring other muscle groups into focus while the ones used previously are resting.

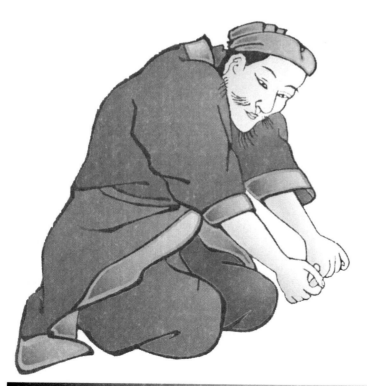

13. Do not give massage with elbow raised above shoulder level

It is quite uncommon for practitioners to find themselves in a position with the elbow over the shoulder level when they are working with a traditional modality at a massage table. However, the advent of chair massage has introduced many new possibilities for losing touch with proper body mechanics. You might find yourself trying to get the leverage that you have become used to achieving during table massage, and in doing so you may lift your elbow up in an attempt to "bear down" from above. Although it may seem like a natural thing to do, working with your elbows raised over your shoulders is not something your body responds favorably to in the long run, nor does it succeed in delivering leverage.

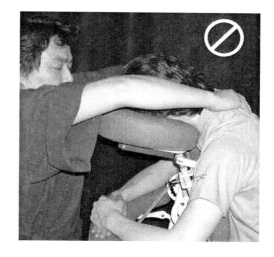

Improper Technique
Working in such a manner that the elbows are rotated outward and are brought above the shoulder joint.

Problem
The angle between the head of the humerus and the glenoid cavity (on the scapula) becomes too acute, weakening the stability of the joint and rendering it both ineffective for deep work and liable to injury.

Proper Technique
When first placing your hand on the client's body, it is acceptable to raise your elbow in order to achieve an optimal hand placement at first. When you are ready to begin the actual application, however, it is important to relax the shoulder and elbow joints, letting the elbow sink toward the ground so that during the application it is beneath the shoulder level.

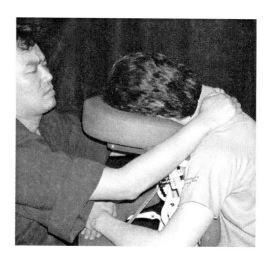

Chapter Three

An Example Routine for Hand Maintenance

As I mentioned earlier, there are many different methods of hand maintenance taught in Japan. I have selected these twenty-five examples of techniques for the arm, wrist, hand, shoulders, and neck. In the professional repertoire there are many more techniques for the arms, shoulders, and hands than are included here, but I have selected these specific techniques because they are the easiest and most effective techniques for the therapist to learn. These techniques, when applied on a consistent basis, help prevent the development of hand pain, cramps, and other irregularities by reducing the tension of the muscles and tendons and increasing the blood and ki flow of the arms and shoulders.

This routine is a method for bringing the precious tools of your trade—your hands, wrists, arms, shoulders, and neck—into optimal working condition for massage therapy. It is not only a method of maintaining strength and flexibility, but it also serves as an excellent preventive measure against injury caused by strain, overwork, and fatigue. This routine is not to be regarded as a way to heal problems that have already developed! Of course, this routine can be used to help existing injuries but that is not the intention of this routine—the point of these exercises is to prevent injuries before they happen. Please understand that preventative measures—not recuperative measures—are the means to a long, healthy career as a massage therapist. If you are careful to combine proper body mechanics at all times and use these hand maintenance exercises before and after massage sessions, you will certainly benefit in the manner of the resilient, rugged Japanese massage-therapists who almost never experience the kinds of hand, wrist, and shoulder problems so commonly found among therapists in the West.

Once the therapist has mastered these techniques, they can easily be modified to apply a very effective treatment for the hands, arms, and shoulders of your clients. You may choose to teach your clients some or all of these simple techniques. They can apply the techniques for everyday care of common ailments, such as carpal tunnel syndrome.

This hand maintenance routine includes techniques for working on the shoulders and neck as well as the hands and forearms. The neck and shoulders are addressed because the nerves and blood vessels for the hands and arms originate there, and these areas (especially the shoulders) are responsible for the origin of many of the movements that the therapist performs when giving a massage. Thus, when the neck and shoulders are relaxed, the therapist has greater mobility and sensitivity in the arms and wrists, which brings about a more fluid massage application. By effectively treating the shoulders and neck, the therapist improves the overall condition of the arms and hands while reducing tension and pain in the upper extremities.

Of course, everybody's hands are different, so modifications may be required to optimize what is best for you. Therefore, it is important for the therapist to understand that the routine I present here is only an example. The therapist may choose to follow this routine exactly or may choose to modify the order in which the techniques are applied to better suit their particular needs. Also, the exact amount of time spent applying these techniques will depend upon the current condition of the therapist's body and the amount of time available to apply these techniques. Some areas of the body may require additional applications to sufficiently warm up the musculature, while other areas may require less time to accomplish the desired results. For example, if you feel tension on the extensor muscles more than anywhere else, you need to pay special attention to this area. By paying such close attention to the needs of your own body and by becoming your own caretaker in this way, you will learn a tremendous amount about your particular problems and how various applications work on your own muscles. Needless to say, this contributes immeasurably to your knowledge, skill, and confidence in your general practice of massage therapy.

Once you become familiar with your hand maintenance routine, **it should take approximately ten minutes to apply all twenty-five techniques.** However, in the beginning it takes longer to complete the routine; take your time and learn how to apply each technique properly. You may find your muscles are sometimes tighter and more tender than usual, particularly the day after you have given many sessions or have done demanding work. If this is the case, take as much time as you need initially to warm the muscles properly. If you need to take twenty minutes, by all means do so. **It is always best to warm your muscles up completely before beginning a day of work.**

Nevertheless, you may sometimes find you do not have the necessary ten minutes to complete the entire routine. In such a case, select a few techniques to warm up the most important regions, such as the hands, forearms, and any especially tight regions, before you work on your first client. You should find a few minutes to apply these techniques before the massage session while your client is undressing or even while you chat with them. It is better to have the client relax on the table for two to three minutes while you are warming up, than to begin a massage without properly warming your body.

To sum up the crucial points of this chapter: warm up extremely well on those days when you feel any tightness, stiffness, or pain. Also, make it a habit to stretch before and after each client, in order to keep your hands and arms loose. An especially important time to apply this routine is the day after a heavy load of massage, in which you may need extra time. Applying this routine daily is an excellent way to maintain your body for a lifetime as a massage therapist.

How to Practice Hand Maintenance Routines

- **Read** each example carefully and slowly until you have a general idea of the procedure and application.
- **Apply** the procedure on yourself for each example, learning them carefully step-by-step according to the instructions. If you are right-handed, use your right hand to apply the technique to your left hand or arm. It is more effective to learn a new technique with your dominant hand first and then later begin to teach your other hand how to do it. However, it is important to actually learn to use your weaker hand, because your dominant hand and arm generally get more use during a massage session and thus need more hand maintenance massage afterward.
- **Connect** the applications together so that they become one fluid routine.
- **Adjust** the routine so that it works best for your needs. You may want to modify the degree of pressure, the length of application, and the number of repetitions of a given technique according to what you need, or you may decide to omit certain techniques that do not seem necessary for you.

When and How Often You Should Apply the Hand Maintenance Routine

It is generally recommended that you apply the routine for ten minutes before your first session of the day. Muscles are tightest in the morning, and it is very important to begin with warm muscles. It is important to do these routines consistently so that tension does not build up over time. For this same reason, it can be very important to give yourself treatment after sessions, as well as at the end of the day if you find it necessary.

What is Necessary for Applying Hand Maintenance Massage?

Nothing special is needed to give excellent treatment. If you have a massage table, you can lay your arm across the massage table and work that way. If you do not have a table, you can work on the floor or on a carpet, pillow, or mat. You can also use a desk or chair (if you are going to work on a hard surface such as wood, metal, or plastic, it is advisable to first lay a folded towel over the surface to provide some cushion on which to work). Although this routine does not require lubrication or oil, it may help when working on the thenar muscle (the pad of the palm).

How Much Pressure Should One Apply for Effective Hand Maintenance?

An excellent quality of self-massage is that you can control the applied pressure perfectly, as you are both the recipient and the therapist. Each example has its own character. Some techniques work well when you apply "almost too much" pressure, while others are most compatible with lighter pressure with a longer duration. Please understand that heavy pressure does not always loosen muscles better; there are definitely situations where muscles respond much better to continual application of lighter pressure.

This Routine Does Not Adequately Replace Massage From Other Qualified Therapists!

Because it is not possible for most therapists to receive hand massage every day from other therapists, we must learn to deliver massage to these areas ourselves so that we can have this therapy every day. Yet, self-massage cannot do everything that regular massage from another professional can do, so we must continue to get professional massages.

Palm Rotation over the Forearms

The purpose of this technique

Reduce tension and increase circulation in the flexor muscles of the forearm and increase mobility of the fingers by separating adhesion between the flexor muscles

Area of application

Over the flexor muscles of the forearm

Description

This technique is good for warming up the forearm. This is one of the most important procedures for hand maintenance, and if you do not have time to do the entire hand maintenance routine, I highly recommend at least doing this technique. It should be applied directly over the flexor digitorum profundus muscle (the deepest of the flexors). This technique improves flexibility of the fingers and reduces the chance of getting carpal tunnel syndrome. This muscle, along with the flexor digitorum superficialis, turns into tendons which go through the carpal tunnels and into the hands; they are also responsible for all hand-flexion movements (such as gripping). The four muscles and tendons of the superficialis are directly on top of the profundus tendons.

Because massage therapists use so much gripping, squeezing, and kneading, it is necessary to strongly work the muscles in the forearm which are responsible for flexing the hand. This technique does not involve sliding over the skin, rather the palm grips the muscle and rotates through the skin into the muscle. If this technique is properly applied, you often feel a slight burning sensation.

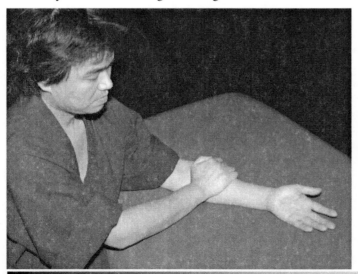

1 Place your left forearm flat on the massage table with your palm facing up. Relax your shoulder, arm, hand, and fingers, allowing them to remain soft. Place the heel of your right hand directly over the flexor muscles of the forearm, just distal to your left elbow, and allow your hand to conform to the contours of the arm. The pads of the fingers may provide support for your hand during the rotation.

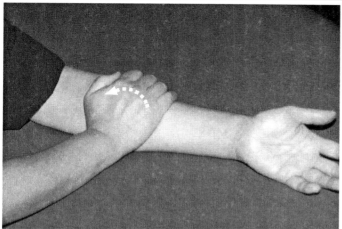

2 Apply firm pressure with the heel of your right hand, hooking into the underlying tissue. Begin to move the heel of your hand in a counterclockwise rotation. Your fingers should bend at the proximal interphalangeal and metacarpophalangeal joints during the application of this technique.

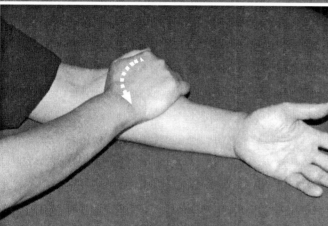

3 A single rotation should take about one second and be continued directly into the next rotation. The diameter of the rotation should be fairly small, as the rotation is determined by the resiliency of the skin on the arm. Remember do not slide over the skin but work through the skin into the underlying muscles. Complete five to ten rotations or as many as desired to effectively warm up the area.

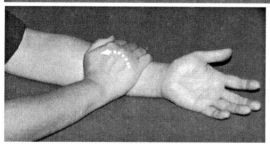

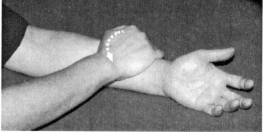

4 Slightly reposition your right hand one inch distal and repeat the procedure. Start with lighter pressure and gradually increase it as the tissue warms up. Once effectively warmed up, this area can withstand a great deal of pressure.

5 Continue to slightly reposition your hand distal and repeat the procedure until the entire flexor side of the forearm has been covered. Reverse your hand and body positions and repeat the entire procedure on your right arm using clockwise rotations with your left hand.

Two-Finger Rotation on the Brachioradialis Muscle

The purpose of this technique

Reduce tension and increase circulation in the brachioradialis

Area of application

Over the anterior portion of the brachioradialis

Description

The brachioradialis, together with the biceps brachii and brachialis, is involved in flexing the elbow, which is one of the most-used areas of movement in massage therapy. Therapists often do not realize how tense this muscle can become. Please note that the brachioradialis originates a few inches above the elbow and extends down to the wrist, with the tendon inserting at the palm.

This example demonstrates two-finger rotation on the brachioradialis. This is another kneading technique, similar to previous movements, but uses two fingers instead of the palm. Cover the entire anterior length of the brachioradialis muscle. With many therapists, the brachioradialis will be sore and tight, especially on those who practice for long periods of time. This technique reduces compression of the elbow joint, which can lead to tendonitis or pain. Because the lung meridian runs along the brachioradialis muscle, including some major acupoints (also known as *tsubo* which are acupressure/acupuncture points), this area and its *tsubo* may be very sensitive (*tsubo* should not be confused with trigger points). The manipulation of these *tsubo* is very useful in reducing tension and pain in this region.

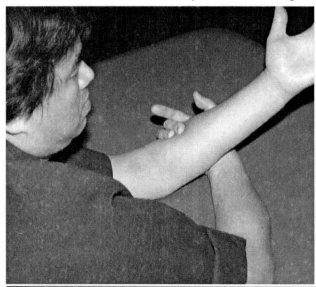

1 Lean against the massage table. Flex your left elbow at 90 degrees to the table, with your forearm straight up in the air and your left palm facing you. Place the heel of your right hand over the extensors of your left forearm, just distal to your elbow. Wrap your ring and middle fingers around the lateral edge of your forearm, placing the pads directly over the medial edge of your left brachioradialis. Your thumb, pinky, and index finger should be relatively straight and should be kept out of the way for this technique.

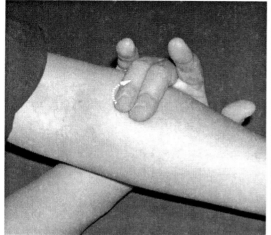

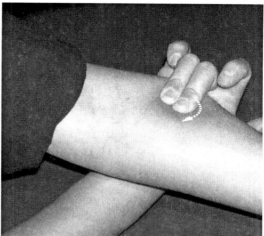

2 Apply pressure with the pads of your ring and middle fingers to compress the tissue against the heel of your hand and hook into the underlying tissue. The heel of the hand acts as a pivot during the rotation. Pull the pads of your fingers in a proximal then lateral direction, gliding over the underlying tissue but not sliding over the skin.

3 Continue to move the pads of your fingers in a distal then medial direction, returning to the starting position. The diameter of the rotation should be about one inch. Complete five to ten rotations or as many as desired. As the area begins to warm up, you may gradually increase the amount of pressure according to your tolerance level.

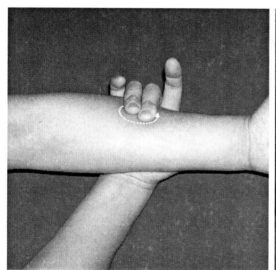

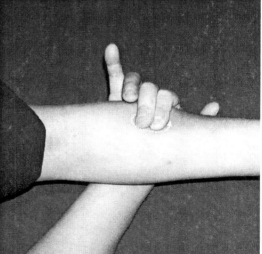

4 Continue to reposition and repeat the procedure until you have covered the entire muscle. You can use your index finger to help reposition your middle and ring finger, resulting in smoother repositioning on the skin.

5 Should you have difficulty using these two fingers, try using the index and middle fingers instead. You may repeat the entire procedure over your forearm as often as necessary. Reverse your hand and body positions, and repeat Steps 1 through 5 on your right forearm.

Hand Maintenance—Example #3

Kneading the Brachioradialis

The purpose of this technique

Reduce tension and increase circulation in the brachioradialis

Area of application

Over the entire brachioradialis

Description

This example is similar to previous examples in which rotation is performed on the brachioradialis to warm up and reduce tension in the muscle.

The kneading movement is one of the most complex movements in massage therapy. These movements are explained in two parts in the following examples. Eventually, these two parts are performed simultaneously and in an alternating fashion, creating a fluid kneading motion which enhances the effectiveness of each technique. Although the entire brachioradialis is kneaded, this technique focuses more on the posterior portion of the brachioradialis. When exercising the brachioradialis, **the wrist of the working hand must remain very loose and flexible.**

Because the Large Intestine Meridian runs along the posterior side of the brachioradialis muscle (which includes some major acupoints—*tsubo*) these *tsubo* may be very sensitive. Again, *tsubo* are not considered trigger points. Stimulation of these *tsubo* is very useful to reduce tension and pain in this region.

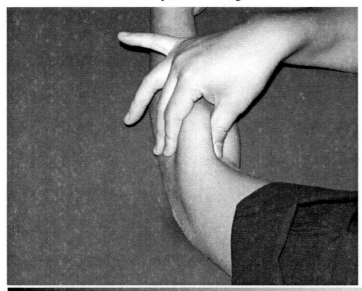

1 Lay your left arm ulnar side down on the massage table, with the elbow relaxed and slightly bent. The arm should be rotated so that the thumb is pointing up. Place the right thumb into the anterior fibers of the brachioradialis, with the pads of the index and middle finger in the posterior fibers. Your right wrist should be slightly above the left arm and should not come in contact with the arm during the procedure.

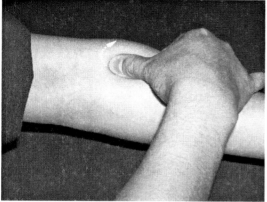
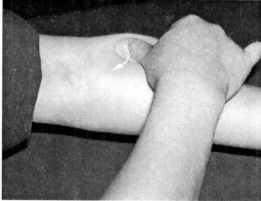

Thumb Rotation on the Anterior Brachioradialis

2 Apply firm pressure with the pads of your thumb, ring, and middle fingers, hooking into the anterior portion of the brachioradialis. Use the pads of the index and middle fingers as a pivot for your hand. Begin to move your thumb in a proximal and then lateral direction. **Your thumb should remain fixed, with the movement originating in your elbow and shoulder. Do not rotate from your thumb joint.**

3 Slowly release the firm pressure with your thumb but remain in contact with the skin of your left forearm as you continue to move your thumb in a distal and then medial direction. Complete ten rotations or as many as desired. Reposition your right hand slightly distal and repeat the rotation. Continue to reposition and repeat the process until the entire muscle has been covered.

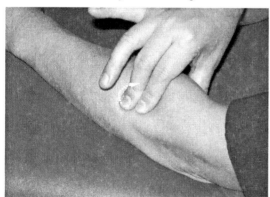
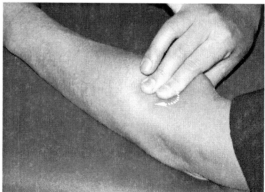

Two-Finger Rotation on the Posterior Brachioradialis

4 Apply firm pressure with the pads of your thumb, index, and middle fingers to hook into the posterior brachioradialis. Alternate between the middle and ring fingers while adjusting the angle of the wrist. Use the pad of your thumb as a pivot for your hand. Pull the pads of your fingers in a proximal and then lateral direction, gliding over the underlying tissue without sliding over your skin.

5 Slowly release the pressure with your fingers but remain in contact with the skin of your left forearm as you continue to move the pads of your fingers in a distal and then medial direction. Complete five to ten rotations or as many as desired. Reposition your right hand slightly distal and repeat, rotating until the entire muscle has been covered. Reverse your hand and body positions repeating Steps 1 through 6 on your right forearm.

Hand Maintenance—Example #4

Percussion on the Forearms

The purpose of this technique

Reduce muscle tension and increase the circulation to the forearms

Area of application

The anterior and posterior sides of the forearms

Description

This example demonstrates percussion on the forearms to increase the circulation to the area and reduce tension in the tissue. This percussion technique is similar to the *tapotement* technique in Swedish massage. There are many different variations of this technique, such as using the back of the hand (see *ANMA: The Art of Japanese Massage*). The effects of this technique depend upon the speed, distance, and stiffness of the wrist during the percussion. **Adjust according to individual sensitivity, and avoid direct hits to the bone.**

Keep the percussion focused over a particular portion of the forearm flexors for a sustained period of time to maximize the effectiveness. Your wrist should be extremely loose when applying percussion.

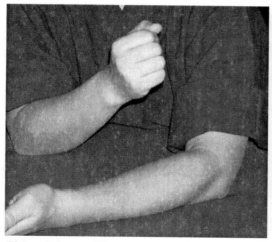 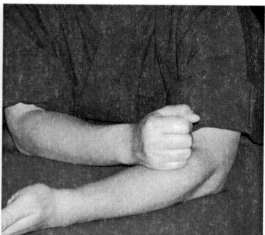

Side of Loose Fist

1 Place your left forearm flat on the massage table with your palm facing up. Relax your shoulder, arm, hand, and fingers, allowing them to remain soft. Make a loose fist with your right hand, keeping enough space between your fingers and palm to fit a Ping-Pong ball. Begin to apply percussion over your left forearm flexors.

2 After stimulating a particular portion of the forearm flexors, reposition your right hand slightly distal to the starting position and repeat until the entire anterior side of the forearm has been sufficiently stimulated.

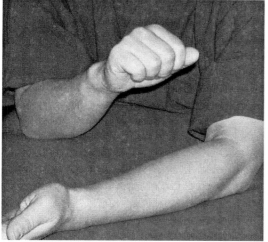

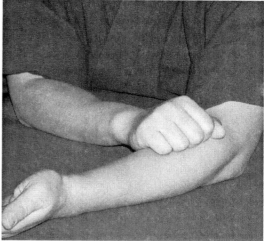

Anterior Surface of Loose Fist

3 Repeat the procedure as described in Steps 1 and 2 except apply the percussion with the posterior surface of your fingers and the anterior surface of the heel of your hand.

4 Pronate your right wrist so the palm is facing your left forearm. Follow the same procedure as before, sustaining your percussion for a little while before slowly repositioning your hand so that the entire muscle is stimulated sufficiently.

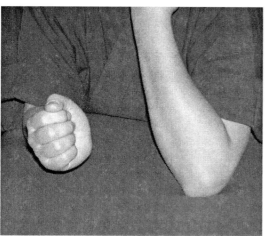

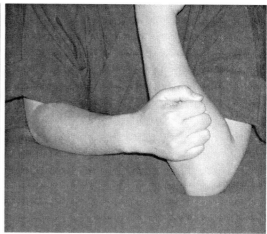

Percussion over the Extensors of the Forearm

5 Flex your left elbow to 45 degrees and place it on the massage table with your forearm angled toward your body. The left palm should be facing your deltoid. Apply percussion with the anterior surface of your loose fist over the extensors of the forearm. Continue for five to ten seconds.

6 Gradually work the percussion up and down the forearm extensors, repositioning your right hand after five or ten seconds. Continue until the entire posterior side of the forearm has been sufficiently stimulated. Reverse your hand and body positions and repeat Steps 1 through 6 over your right forearm.

Thumb Pressure on the Radius and Ulna

The purpose of this technique

Reduce muscle tension and increase energy (*ki*) flow in the anterior forearm

Area of application

On the anterior forearm

Description

This example demonstrates light, fluid pressure over the flexors of the forearm with your thumb to reduce muscular tension. Increased energy (*ki*) flow in the forearm is essential for maintenance of the hand as well as to give quality treatment.

There are six channels (*keiraku* or meridians) of energy that flow through the hand, and in each one, energy is driven from different internal organs. Three *yin* channels flow from the chest to the fingertips. Three *yang* channels flow from the fingertips, through the shoulders, and into the face. For more information on *ki* and meridians, refer to *ANMA: The Art of Japanese Massage.*

While you are giving self-massage on the anterior forearm, it may be easier to apply the technique from the wrist to the elbow. You may go in opposite directions to follow the flow of the *ki*, by applying pressure from the elbow to the wrist, once you get used to applying fluid pressure. The application of fluid pressure is common in anma or shiatsu, and it is useful when used in conjunction with other massage modalities.

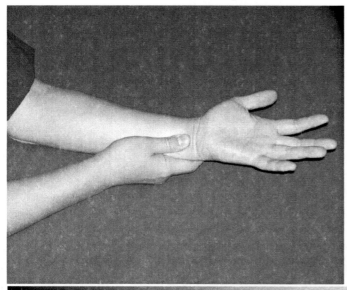

1 Lay your left forearm flat on the massage table with your palm facing up. Slide the fingers from your right hand under your left forearm, with your right palm facing up. Place the pad of your right thumb directly over the medial edge of your left ulna, just proximal to the wrist.

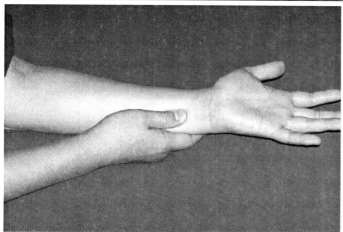

2 Apply light pressure with your right thumb, hooking into the underlying tissue. Gently push your thumb toward your wrist, stroking about one half-inch.

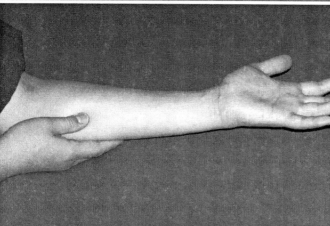

3 Lightly slide your thumb proximally past the starting position. Gently push your thumb as before. Each time you reposition your thumb, place it so that the ending point of the next stroke overlaps with the starting position of the previous stroke. Continue to repeat the procedure until you have covered the entire ulna.

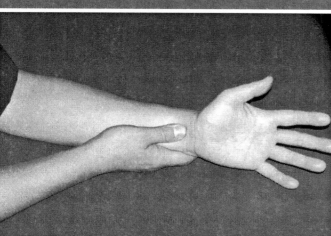

4 Reposition your thumb to apply the technique between the radius and ulna, repeating Steps 2 and 3. Then, reposition your thumb again while rotating the left hand slightly to better accommodate the action. Apply the technique over the lateral edge of your left radius. Reverse your hand and body positions and repeat the entire procedure over your right forearm, with your left hand.

Two-Finger Rotation on the Posterior Forearm

The purpose of this technique

Reduce muscle tension and increase energy (*ki*) flow in the posterior forearm

Area of application

Over the posterior side of the forearm

Description

This example demonstrates two-finger rotation over the extensor side of the forearm. The extensor muscles are another group used heavily by therapists. To relieve soreness, thoroughly work the extensors. Use the index and middle fingers of your right hand to apply the two-finger rotation. Slightly overlap your index over your middle finger (you can also alternate your middle and ring finger to avoid fatigue) to provide some additional support for your fingers during the rotation.

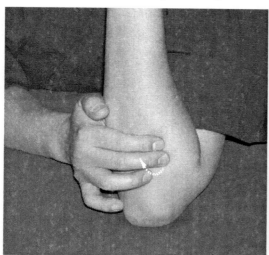
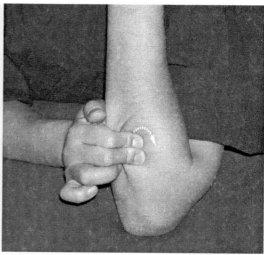

1 Place your left arm on the massage table. Flex your elbow so the forearm is nearly vertical and relax your wrist. Place the pads of your right index and middle fingers over the extensor side of your left forearm, just distal to your elbow between the lateral edge of your radius bone and the posterior edge of your brachioradialis. Place the thenar side of the heel of your right hand over the medial portion of your left forearm flexors to act as a pivot for your hand during the rotation.

2 Apply firm pressure with the pads of your index and middle fingers to hook into the tissue. Using the thenar side of your hand as a pivot, apply small rotations with the pads of your fingers. The diameter of the rotations should be about one inch. Complete five to ten rotations or as many as desired. Reposition your fingers slightly distal, following the lateral edge of your left radius bone and repeat the rotations. Continue to reposition your fingers, repeating the procedure until you reach your wrist.

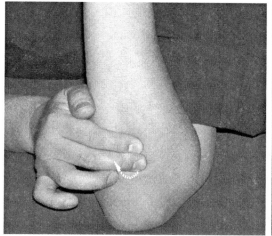

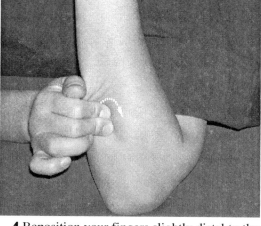

3 Reposition your fingers between your ulna and radius, just distal to your elbow. Place the pad of your thumb over the flexors to act as a pivot during the rotation. Apply pressure with the pads of your index and middle fingers to hook into the tissue. Apply small rotations with the pads of your fingers. Complete five to ten rotations or as many as desired.

4 Reposition your fingers slightly distal to the starting point, following the medial edge of your left radius bone, and repeat the rotation. Continue to reposition your fingers and repeat the procedure until you reach your wrist. You may repeat the rotation over the same region as necessary.

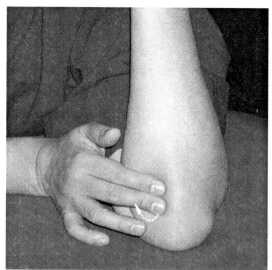

5 This is the same procedure as described in Steps 3 and 4, except the fingers should be positioned at the medial edge of the ulna, just distal to your elbow. Place the pad of your thumb over the flexors to act as a pivot for the rotation. Apply small rotations as in Steps 3 and 4.

6 Reposition your fingers slightly distal, following the medial edge of your left ulna, and repeat the rotation. Reverse your hand and body positions, and repeat Steps 1 through 6 over your right forearm.

Hand Maintenance—Example #7

Rotation over the Wrist

The purpose of this technique

Reduce tension in the wrist, which increases strength and flexibility and prevents injury in the wrist during massage

Area of application

Both the dorsal and palmar sides of the wrist

Description

This example demonstrates thumb and two-finger rotation over the wrist joint. Apply light, even pressure. Overall, better results are achieved by using **sustained, light pressure** rather than deeper application into the wrist joint, which can aggravate wrist problems. The focus of this technique is to warm the entire wrist area and create more flexibility.

Do not rotate the thumb from the carpometacarpal, or metacarpophalangeal joint. The hand should move as a unit. This is a good technique to practice until the biomechanical action becomes second nature.

Slightly adjust the angle of your wrist, extending it in the opposite direction of the application. This exposes the area of application and increases the effectiveness of the procedure.

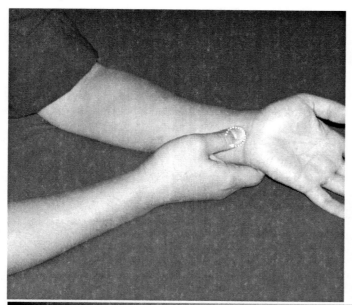

Thumb Rotation on Anterior Wrist

1 Lay your left forearm on the massage table with your palm facing up. Place the pad of your right thumb just proximal to the hypothenar side of the wrist joint. Gently wrap the fingers of your right hand under your left forearm to support and stabilize your hand. Apply light pressure with your right thumb to hook into the underlying tissue. Begin to move the pad of your thumb in small clockwise circles, with the movement coming from your elbow, as your entire hand moves as a unit. **Do not rotate from your thumb joint.**

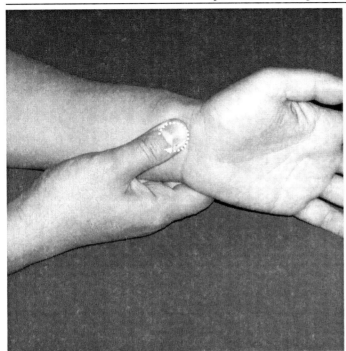

2 Continue to apply rotation for three to five seconds or as long as desired. Reposition your thumb laterally about one half-inch and repeat the rotation. You may pronate your forearm as you reposition your thumb to maintain proper alignment of the thumb.

Two-Finger Rotation on the Posterior Wrist

3 For the posterior side of your left wrist, place the lower portion of the right palm against the anterior side of the left wrist. Place the tips of the middle and ring finger into the wrist joint, between the radius, ulna, and carpal bones. Apply gentle pressure with the tips of the right fingers, making small, clockwise rotations with the heel of the hand. Repeat for five to ten rotations. Reverse your hand and body positions, repeating the entire procedure on your right wrist and using your left fingers to apply counterclockwise rotations.

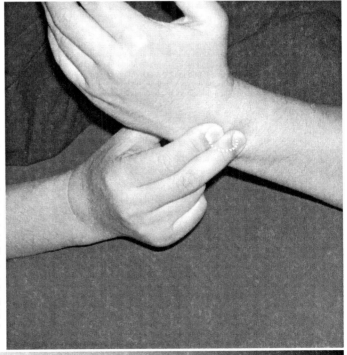

Fascial Release on the Wrist

The purpose of this technique

Reduce fascial adhesion and improve the range of motion in the wrist

Area of application

At the base of the hand on both sides of the forearm

Description

This example demonstrates fascial release techniques for your wrists. Fascia is the thin, tough connective tissue that encases muscles and organs in the body. Adhesion of the skin or muscle to the fascial layers restricts movement of the wrist and hand. Frequent release of fascial adhesion not only prevents injury but also increases flexibility, promoting smoother movements during massage.

This fascial release technique is accomplished by applying pressure with your thumb into your forearm to trap the underlying tissue and fascia and then to take your wrist through a specific range of motion to stretch the fascia. For example, if you wish to stretch the fascia on the posterior side of your forearm, trap the posterior side and then very slowly flex your wrist. The direction in which you move your wrist is opposite of the specific area trapped with either your fingers or thumb.

When properly stretching the fascia, you should feel a burning sensation during the application. If you extend your wrist too quickly, you are not properly stretching the fascia. This technique only needs to be repeated once or twice. You can also perform fascial techniques on both the medial and lateral sides of the wrist, which may improve the range of abduction and adduction in the wrist.

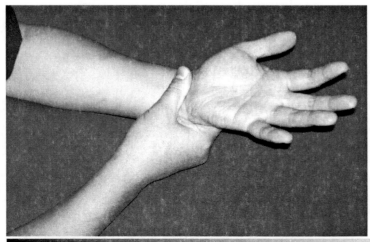

1 Place your left elbow on the massage table with your forearm slightly elevated off the table, your wrist in the neutral position and your palm facing up. Place the four fingers of your right hand over the posterior side of your left forearm, just proximal to your wrist joint. Place your right thumb over the anterior side of the forearm, perpendicular to the ulna and radius and just proximal to the wrist joint.

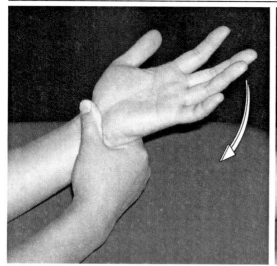

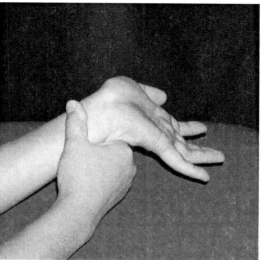

2 Apply very firm pressure with your right thumb into the anterior side of your forearm to trap the underlying tissue and fascia.

3 **Very slowly** extend your wrist to the end of your range of motion, while applying very firm pressure with the thumb. You will know that the fascia is being stretched effectively when you feel a burning sensation. Repeat one more time if necessary.

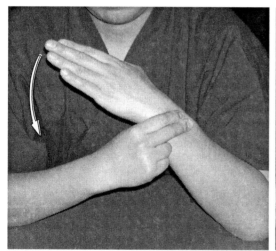

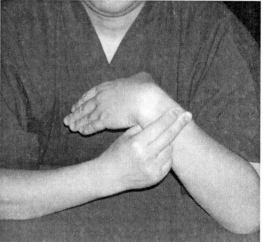

4 Place the pads of the index and middle fingers of your right hand firmly into the posterior side of your left wrist, between the heads of the radius and ulna, in a 45 degree angle to the surface of the wrist. Place your right thumb over the anterior side of your wrist, as in Step 2.

5 Apply very firm pressure with your right thumb into the posterior side of your forearm to trap the underlying tissue and fascia. **Very slowly** flex your wrist to the end of your range of motion. Repeat the stretch two to three times or as many times as desired. Reverse your hand and body positions and repeat Steps 1 through 5 to your right wrist.

Deep Rotation on the Muscles of the Palm

The purpose of this technique

Reduce tension in the muscles of the palms

Area of application

Over the thenar and hypothenar muscles of the palms

Description

This example demonstrates deep rotation over the muscles of the palms. The muscles that are focused upon on the thenar side are the abductor pollicis brevis and opponens pollicis muscles. On the hypothenar side, the abductor digitorum minimi and opponens digitorum minimi muscles are covered. If you use your thumb frequently or use applications with finger manipulation in general, such as facial or foot massage, the thenar/hypothenar muscles tend to become over worked. Maintenance is very important for these muscles to relieve tightness or soreness and to keep them in good working order.

Whether using two-finger or thumb rotation, the pivot point should stem from the entire hand. **Do not rotate from the carpometacarpal, or metacarpophalangeal joint.** The wrist should always be loose enough to accommodate the entire movement.

Although there are many different techniques to work the thenar and hypothenar muscles, the example here works the muscle of the hand most effectively and evenly to release muscular tension.

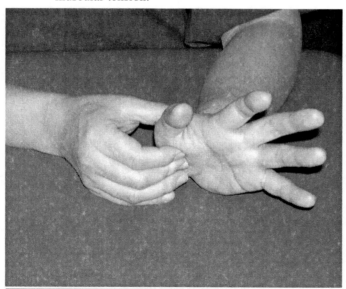

Two-Finger Rotation on the Thenar Muscles

1 Place your left elbow on the massage table, with your forearm slightly elevated off the table and your palm facing down. Slightly overlap the pads of your index and middle fingers, placing them over the thenar side of your left palm. Place the pad of your right thumb over the posterior surface of your first and second metacarpal to act as a pivot for your hand during the rotation.

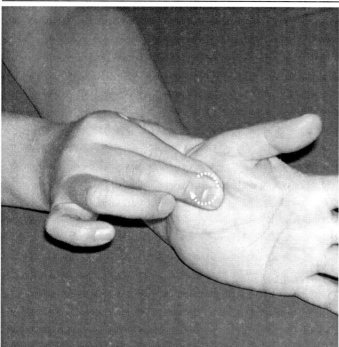

2 Overlap the pads of the index and middle fingers and apply firm pressure, hooking into the underlying tissue. Begin to rotate the pads of your fingers in small circles. **Glide over the underlying tissue and do not slide over your skin.** Apply the rotation for five to ten seconds or as long as desired. Continue to reposition your fingers and repeat the procedure until the entire thenar muscle has been covered.

Thumb Rotation on the Hypo-thenar Muscles

3 Reposition to apply rotation over the hypothenar side of your palm. Place the pad of your right thumb just proximal to the hypothenar muscles. Place the fingers of your right hand over the fifth metacarpal to stabilize and support your hand. Apply light pressure with your right thumb, hooking into the underlying tissue. Begin to move the pad of your thumb in small clockwise circles, with the movement coming from your elbow. **Do not rotate from your thumb joint.** Apply the rotation for five to ten seconds or as long as desired. Continue to reposition your fingers and repeat the procedure until the entire hypothenar muscle has been covered. Reverse your hand and body positions and repeat the procedure on the right hand.

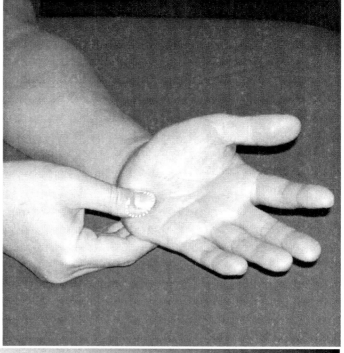

Stroking between the Metacarpals with the Thumbs

The purpose of this technique

Reduce tension in the muscles between the metacarpals

Area of application

Between the metacarpals of the hands

Description

This example demonstrates thumb stroking between the metacarpals. **The thumb should not be bent or hyperabducted while stroking. It should be pointed in the direction of the stroke during this technique.** You should not require the use of any lubricant to perform this technique properly, but if you feel the skin being pulled while stroking, you may use a minimal amount of lotion to lessen the friction.

It is best to stroke in the direction of energy (*ki*) flow. On the palmar side, stroke toward the fingertips. On the dorsal side, stroke from the fingertips toward the wrist.

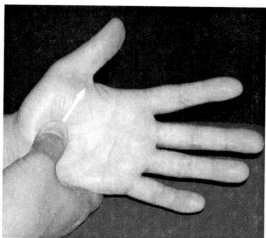
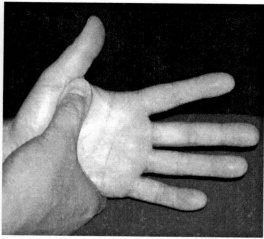

1 Lay your left forearm flat on the massage table with your hand slightly elevated off the table. Place the anterior surface of the fingers of your right hand underneath your left hand. Place the pad of your thumb between your left first and second metacarpal bones, just distal to your thumb and carpometacarpal joint. Apply firm pressure with your right thumb and stroke lateral direction between the first and second metacarpals, following the medial edge of your first metacarpal bone.

2 Once you reach the edge of the web, release the pressure and return to your starting position. Repeat the stroking three to five times or as many times as desired. Gradually alter the direction of your stroking from a lateral to distal direction, covering the space between the first and second metacarpal bones. Reposition your right thumb between your second and third metacarpal bones and repeat the stroke. Stay between the bones while stroking.

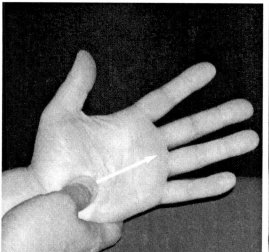

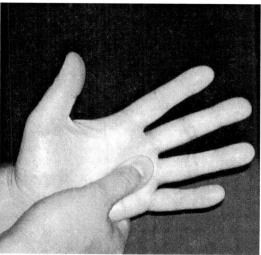

3 Reposition your right thumb between the third and fourth metacarpal bones and repeat the stroking three to five times or as many times as desired.

4 Again, reposition your right thumb between the fourth and fifth metacarpal bones and repeat the stroking three to five times or as many times as desired. You may repeat Steps 1 through 5 as many times as necessary.

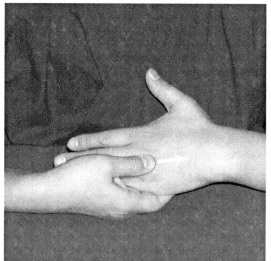

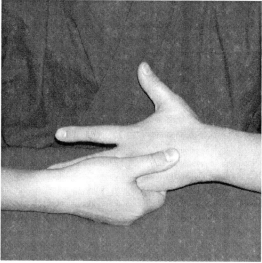

5 To work the dorsal side of your left hand, pronate your left wrist, placing the forefingers of the right hand over the medial side of the left palm. Place the thumb between the fourth and fifth metacarpophalangeal joints and begin stroking between the fourth and fifth metacarpals until you reach the carpal bones. Stroke slowly on the posterior side of your hand.

6 Reposition and repeat the stroking between each metacarpal bone until the dorsal side has been sufficiently covered. Reverse your hand and body positions, repeating Steps 1 through 6 on your right hand. The posterior side tends to be drier than the anterior side so you may need to apply a drop of lotion.

Massage around *Go Koku*

The purpose of this technique

Reduce tension and relieve fatigue in the thenar muscles

Area of application

Over the muscles between the first and second metacarpals

Description

This example demonstrates kneading the muscles between the first and second metacarpal bones, specifically the adductor pollicis, flexor pollicis brevis, and abductor pollicis brevis muscles. Pressure and massage applied around the *go koku* (Large Intestine-4) helps reduce tension in the thenar muscles and surrounding area, as well as relieving headaches and shoulder tension while increasing blood and *ki* flow to the hand. **It is very important to avoid working this point during the first and second trimester of pregnancy.**

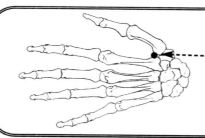

合谷

Go koku—**Large Intestine-4**
(*ho ku*; Chinese pronunciation)
The location of *go koku* is the junction between the first and second metacarpals on the dorsal side. You can find an indentation on the base of the second metacarpal, over the the dorsal metacarpal ligament.

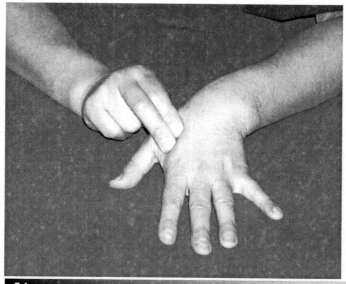

1 Place your left elbow, flexed to 45 degrees, on the massage table with your hand elevated six inches off the table and the palm facing down. Place the pads of your right index and middle fingers over the muscles between the first and second metacarpal bones, on the posterior side of your left hand. Place the pad of your right thumb on the muscles between the first and second metacarpal bones, on the anterior side of your left hand. Your thumb should be directly opposite the pads of your index and middle fingers.

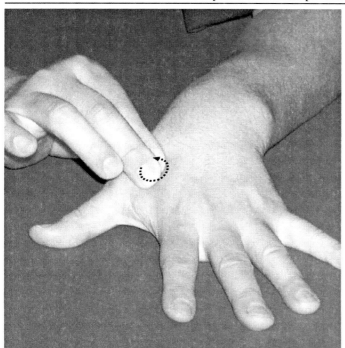

2 Apply light pressure with the pads of your thumb, index, and middle fingers to hook into the underlying tissue. Using your thumb as a pivot, rotate your index and middle fingers in small circles. The index and middle finger should overlap, with the pressure being driven through the index finger. Make a habit of overlapping your fingers during rotation to offer support and minimize undue stress to the working fingers. Complete five to seven rotations or as many as desired. Gradually increase the amount of pressure after the tissue has been sufficiently warmed up.

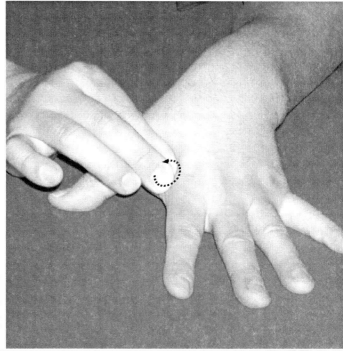

3 Slightly reposition your fingers and repeat the procedure. Continue to repeat the process until the entire area in between the first and second metacarpal bones has been covered. Then reverse your hand and body positions and repeat Steps 1 through 3 on your right hand.

Light Stroking on the Fingers

The purpose of this technique

Increase circulation while lightly stretching the fingers

Area of application

Over the anterior and posterior surface of the fingers

Description

This example is very similar to Example #10 but demonstrates stroking over the fingers and thumbs. Again, it is best to stroke in the direction of the energetic (*ki*) flow. On the palmar side, stroke toward the fingertips. On the dorsal side, stroke from the fingertips toward the wrist.

This technique can be very helpful for therapists with poor finger circulation or hands that are often cold, which from the Asian therapeutic perspective indicates that there is a *ki* flow impediment. This situation can affect the energetic relationship between therapist and client. Warming the hands greatly increases the therapeutic value and overall results of your massage.

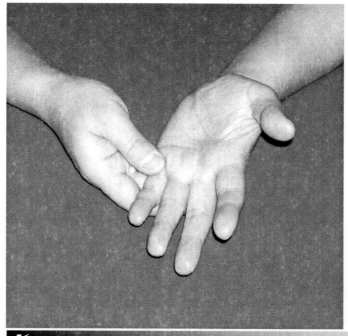

1 Place your left elbow on the massage table with the palm facing up. **Always place the four fingers of the working hand under the finger of the receiving hand to support the finger and prevent hyperextension.**

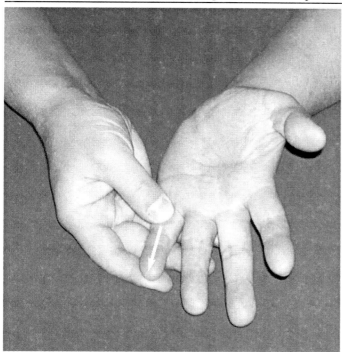

2 Place the pad of your right thumb over your left pinky, just distal to the metacarpophalangeal joint. Apply light pressure into your pinky with your right thumb, gently sliding your thumb toward the tip until you reach the end of your left pinky.

3 Release the light pressure and bring your thumb back again, while still remaining in contact with the pinky. The initial stroke applies greater pressure than the return stroke. Repeat the stroking for three to five seconds, or as long as desired, to warm up the finger. Reposition your right thumb to stroke your ring finger. Adjust the four fingers of your right hand to support your left ring finger and prevent hyperextension. Continue to reposition, and repeat the technique on all four fingers.

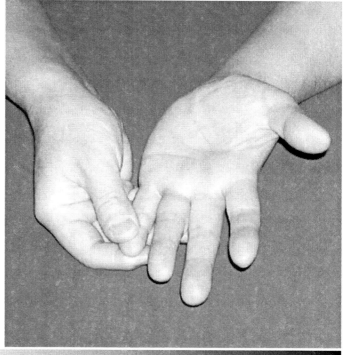

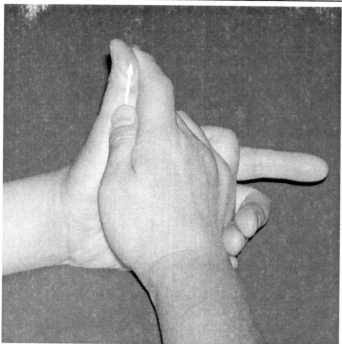

4 Reposition your right thumb just distal to the metacarpopha-langeal joint of your left thumb. Stroke to the end of your left thumb, maintaining even pressure throughout the entire stroke.

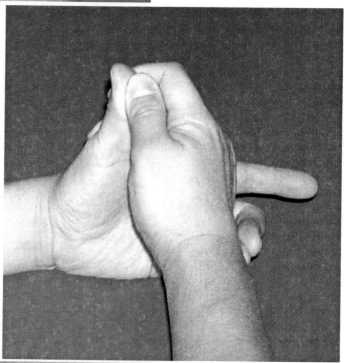

5 Reverse your stroke and return to the starting position. Repeat the stroking for three to five seconds or as long as desired.

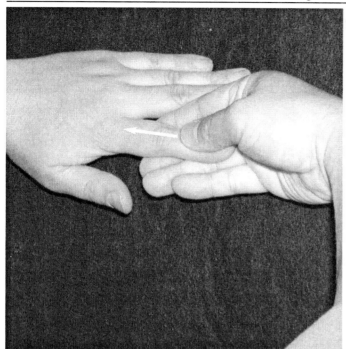

6 Pronate your wrist so that palm is facing down. Repeat the same procedure over the dorsal surface of your fingers and thumb. Stroke from the fingertip, across the nail bed, and toward the metacarpophalangeal joint. **Be sure to support the left fingers with the four fingers of your right hand as you apply the technique.** Although you can stroke distally, it is recommended to work in the direction of the *ki* flow.

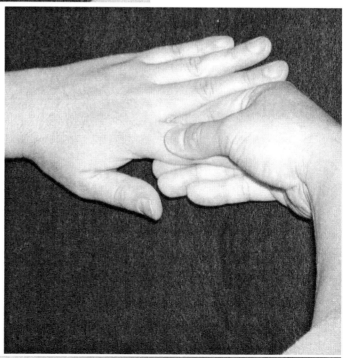

7 Repeat the procedure on the rest of the fingers, then reverse your hand and body positions and repeat Steps 1 through 3 on your right hand.

Thumb Rotation on the Joints of the Fingers

The purpose of this technique

Reduce tension and increase fluid circulation in the joints of the fingers

Area of application

Over the posterior and anterior surface of the fingers

Description

This example demonstrates rotation on the fingers to reduce tension, prevent joint aches, and increase circulation in the joints. You can also rotate between the pads and joints of the fingers. Apply light, even pressure, which is often more effective than vigorous, deep pressure. You can rotate the fingers of the receiving hand slightly to cover the side of the phalangeal joint. **The four fingers of the giving hand should support the finger of the receiving hand.**

When learning, and later while practicing this technique, be sure to have the action stem from the entire hand, rather than the carpometacarpal or metacarpophalangeal joints. Even while working with very light pressure, focus on biomechanics to prevent muscular fatigue within the thenar joint.

This technique, when used in conjunction with others shown in this book and slightly modified, can be very useful for clients who have joint pain, such as arthritis.

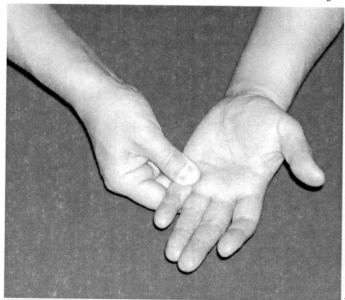

1 Place your left elbow flexed on the massage table. Your palm should be facing up and slightly above the table surface. Place the pads of your right four fingers underneath your left pinky to support it while applying the rotation. Place the pad of your right thumb over the metacarpophalangeal joint of your left pinky.

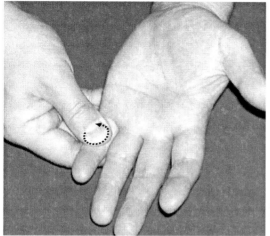

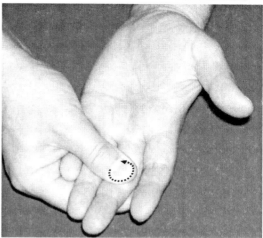

2 With your right thumb, apply light pressure into your left pinky and rotate your thumb in very small circles. The movement should come from your right wrist and shoulder. Try to keep your thumb as fixed as possible. Apply the rotation for three to five seconds, moving your thumb from the proximal interphalangeal joint distally.

3 Continue the procedure on the distal interphalangeal joint on the pinky, then reposition your thumb onto your ring finger and repeat. Continue to reposition and repeat the procedure until all four fingers and the thumb have been covered. If desired, you can work on the thumb joint.

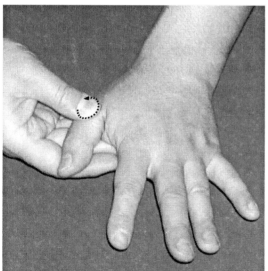

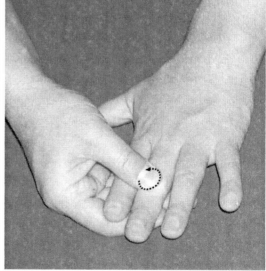

4 Pronate your wrist so the palm is facing down. Apply the same procedure over the posterior surface of your fingers and thumb.

5 **When applying this technique, support each finger as you apply the technique with the four fingers of your right hand.** Reverse your hand and body positions, repeating Steps 1 through 5 on your right hand.

Hand Maintenance—Example #14

Traction and Decompression of the Fingers

The purpose of this technique

Stretch and decompress the joints of the fingers

Area of application

On the fingers

Description

The next four examples demonstrate stretching techniques on the wrists, hands, and fingers. This technique has the same effects as light stroking over the fingers (see Example #12). Should you have time constraints, this may be supplemented for both techniques.

Although often misunderstood, effective anatomical stretching occurs in conjunction with respiration (stretching occurs during exhalation) and the extension of joints **slightly** beyond the normal range of motion (R.O.M.). Extend only slightly beyond the normal R.O.M. Do not hold the stretch longer than the length of one full exhalation. Muscle fiber damage can occur if you hold the stretch for over thirty seconds. When moving the joint through its R.O.M., there is often some sound produced from the natural release of stored gases (the same sound you hear when you "crack" your knuckles). Although this is naturally occurring, it should not be the focus of the action.

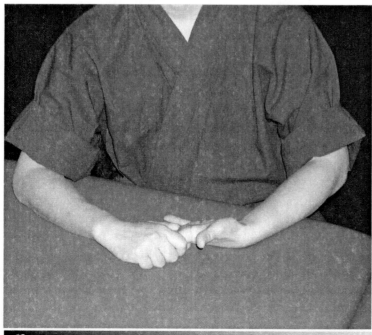

1 Place your left elbow on the massage table, with your elbow flexed at 45 degrees and your hand raised slightly above the table with the palm facing up. Lightly grasp your left index finger with your right hand, just distal to the metacarpophalangeal joint.

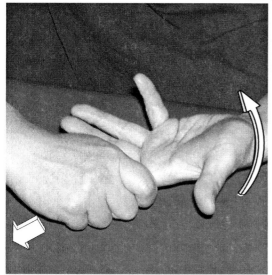

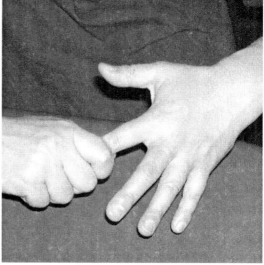

2 Pull your left index finger straight out with enough pressure so the right hand begins to slide over your index finger. You may incorporate a slight twisting movement while you are pulling the finger.

3 You should not require any lubrication to effectively apply this technique. Repeat the process two to three times or as many times as desired.

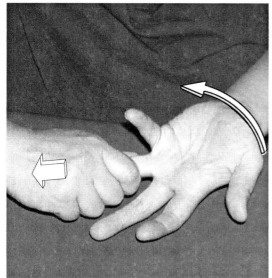

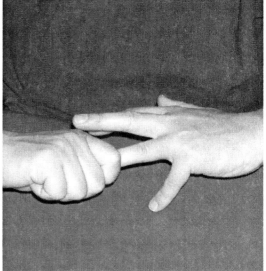

4 Release the index finger, repositioning your right hand to apply the technique to your left middle finger. Repeat the same procedure for each of your fingers.

5 **You may also perform this technique on your thumb, but do not incorporate any twisting movement.** Reverse your hand and body positions and repeat Steps 1 through 5 on your right hand.

Interlocking and Stretching the Fingers

The purpose of this technique

Decompress the flexors and metacarpophalangeal joint of the hand

Area of application

On the metacarpophalangeal joints of both hands

Description

This example demonstrates a stretching technique for the metacarpophalangeal joints; it is a very important technique for keeping the joints healthy and properly functioning. In this application, move very smoothly and slowly while exhaling. A bad habit that many therapists have is the simultaneous stretching of both hands from an interlocked position. This stretch should be avoided, especially by people who use the fingers repetitively, as in massage, piano, guitar, etc.

Do not stretch both hands at the same time

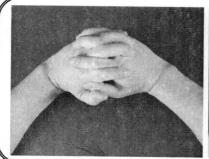 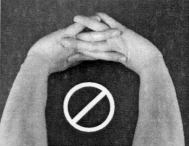

Do not stretch both hands at the same time. This may overstretch both hands, possibly hyperextend the joints of your fingers, and cause soft tissue and joint damage.

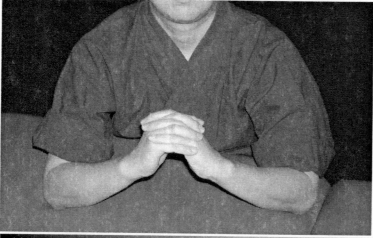

1 Loosely interlace your fingers and position the pads of the fingers of your right hand over the metacarpophalangeal joints of your left hand. Your left hand should be soft and relaxed.

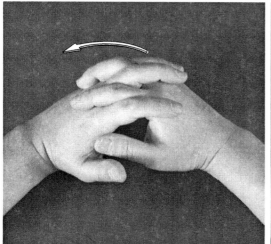

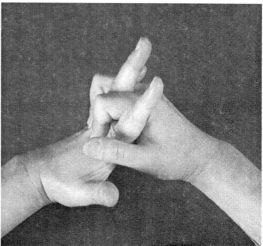

2 Begin to apply pressure with the pads of your fingers into the metacarpophalangeal joints of the fingers of your left hand. The fingers of your right hand should be flexed about 90 degrees at the proximal interphalangeal joints and **slightly** hyperextended at the distal interphalangeal joints.

3 With the application of pressure from your right hand, the metacarpophalangeal joints of the fingers of your left hand should slightly hyperextend. Hold the stretch for three to five seconds and release. **Do not overstretch your hand and fingers or you may cause damage to the tissue.**

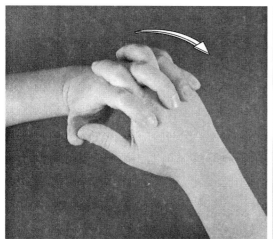

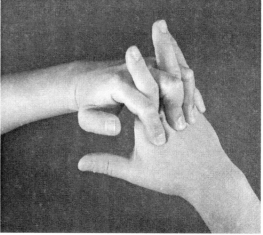

4 Reverse your hand and finger positions so the pads of the fingers of your left hand are over the metacarpophalangeal joints of the fingers of your right hand. Your right hand should be soft and relaxed. Begin to apply pressure with the pads of your fingers into the metacarpophalangeal joints of the fingers of your right hand. Repeat Steps 2 and 3 on the right hand.

5 Hold the stretch for three to five seconds and release. Continue stretching each hand. While alternating between the two, increase the depth of the stretch with each repetition. Be sure to **slightly** extend—not excessively hyperextend—the joints in this technique.

Gentle Stretching of the Wrist

The purpose of this technique

Stretch the wrist, improving flexibility and preventing injury

Area of application

On the hands and wrist

Description

This example demonstrates stretching techniques for your hands and wrists. As in the previous example, stretching should slightly exceed the normal R.O.M.. Do not force the stretch, especially on the wrist, or hold for too long. By incorporating slow, controlled exhalation, the benefits of this stretch are greatly increased.

If you feel any pain or discomfort when applying this stretching technique, you should return to loosening the flexors and extensors (Examples #1 and #6). Try loosening with rotation of the wrist (Example #7), and you can also try stretching the wrist by pulling the hand straight away from the arm for ten seconds and then gently releasing. Repeat five to ten times and then attempt the stretch in this example. If you still have pain or discomfort, refrain from using this technique.

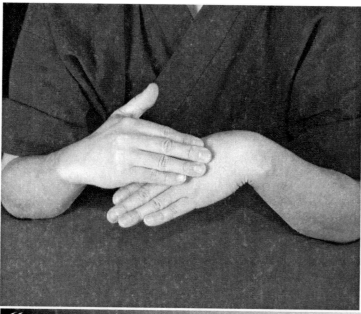

Flexion of the Wrist

1 Place your left arm on the massage table. Flex your left elbow and wrist about 90 degrees so the forearm is relatively vertical and the palm of your left hand is facing down. Place the anterior surface of the fingers of your right hand over the posterior surface of your left hand. Your left hand, wrist, and forearm should be soft and relaxed.

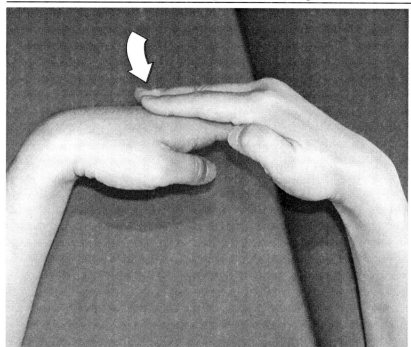

2 Apply **gentle** pressure with your right hand into the posterior surface of your left hand to stretch the posterior portion of your left wrist gently. **Do not overstretch your wrist.**

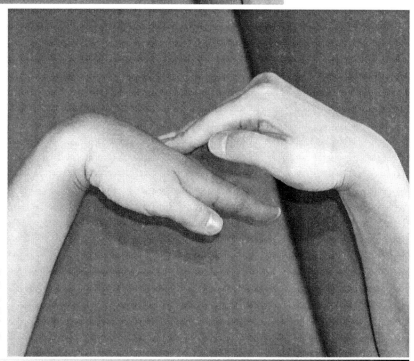

3 Hold the stretch for five to seven seconds and release. Repeat the stretch two to three times or as many times as desired.

Extension of the Wrist

4 Use a similar starting position as described in Step 1 except extend your wrist about 90 degrees from the neutral position and place the anterior surface of the fingers of your right hand over the palm of your left hand. Apply light pressure with your right hand into the palm of your left hand to gently stretch the anterior portion of your left wrist. **Do not overstretch your wrist.** Hold the stretch for five to seven seconds, while exhaling, and then release. Repeat the stretch two to three times or as many times as desired. Reverse your hand and body positions, and repeat the stretching procedure on your right wrist.

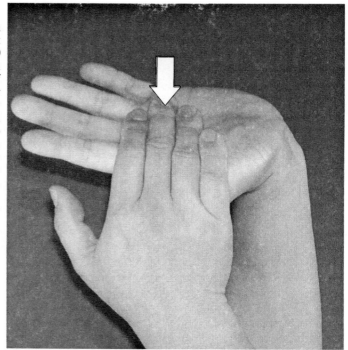

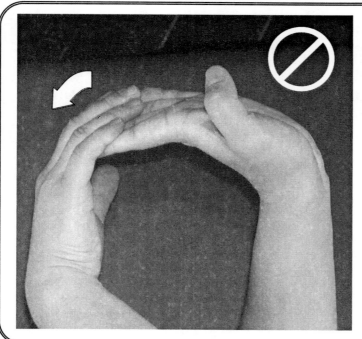

Do not place your right hand over the anterior surface of your left fingers to stretch your left hand. This hyperextends the fingers and wrist, causing undue stress and strain on your joints.

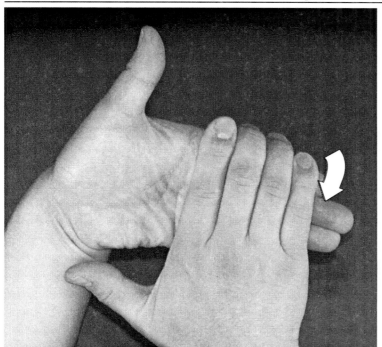

Adduction of the Wrist

5 Place the right fingers along the medial edge of the left hand. With the forearm and wrist stabilized, bring the right hand toward you and stretch while exhaling. **Do not overstretch your wrist.** Hold the stretch for five to seven seconds while exhaling and then release. Repeat the stretch two to three times or as many times as desired. Reverse your hand and body positions and repeat the stretching procedure on your right wrist.

Abduction of the Wrist

6 Place the forearm directly over the massage table with the wrist over the edge. Place the four fingers of the right hand over the first metacarpal of the left hand. Apply light pressure with your right hand into the first metacarpal of your left hand to gently stretch the lateral portion of your left wrist. **Do not overstretch your wrist.** Hold the stretch for five to seven seconds while exhaling and then release. Repeat the stretch two to three times or as many times as desired. Reverse your hand and body positions and repeat the stretching procedure on your right wrist.

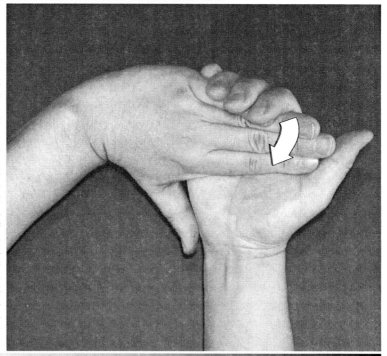

Stretching between the Metacarpals by Compressing the Palm

The purpose of this technique

Increase flexibility and reduce tension in the metacarpals

Area of application

On the hands

Description

This example demonstrates stretching by compression of the hand to reduce tension and increase the flexibility between the metacarpals. If you feel very tight and inflexible between the metacarpals, combine stroking the metacarpals with the thumb (Example #10) with this stretching technique, which improves flexibility and creates fluid movement between the metacarpals. This is essential for keeping the hands in optimal condition.

As with the previous example, apply while exhaling. **Do not use excessive force during this stretch.** Should severe pain or discomfort occur, avoid this technique.

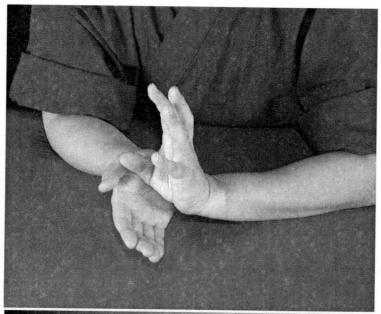

1 Place your left arm on the massage table. Flex your left elbow about 90 degrees so the forearm is relatively vertical. When you are comfortable with this technique, the hand can be lowered to a level plane. Place the heel of your right hand over the lateral portion of your left thumb's metacarpal bone.

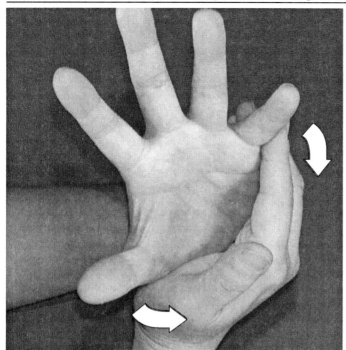

2 Place the pads of the fingers of your right hand over the medial side of your left hand. Your left hand should be soft and relaxed during the application of this example.

3 Apply firm pressure with the pads of your fingers and with the heel of your right hand to compress your left hand. Hold the compression for three to five seconds and release. Repeat the compression two to three times or as many times as desired. Reverse your hand and body positions and repeat the procedure on your right hand.

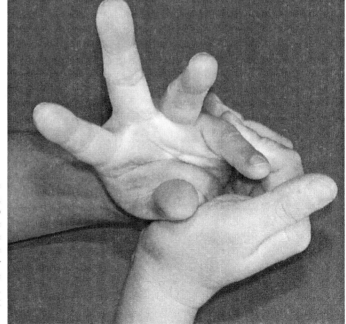

Pressure and Rotation on the Carpal Ligaments

The purpose of this technique

Reduce tension and increase flexibility in the carpal ligaments

Area of application

Directly over the flexor retinaculum

Description

This example demonstrates deep thumb pressure and thumb rotation over the carpal ligaments. The purpose of this technique is to stretch the carpal ligaments, reducing the compression and stress in the carpal tunnel. This allows smoother movement of the flexors under the flexor retinaculum.

This technique is mainly for Western massage therapists and other therapists who repetitively use the flexors. Anma (Japanese massage therapy) practitioners never have carpal tunnel syndrome, because self-maintenance is an inherent product of the practice. For example, using palm rotation as a general therapeutic movement on the client simultaneously acts as a hand/carpal technique of considerable therapeutic value for the practitioner that loosens the flexors of the forearm and reduces stress in the carpal tunnel. This technique is therefore a very effective way to treat clients who are suffering from carpal tunnel syndrome.

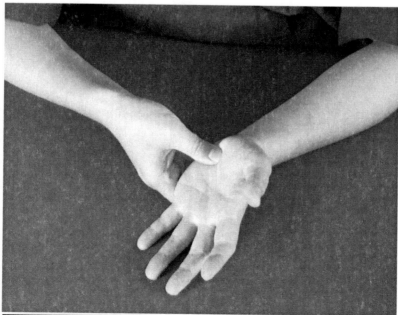

1 Place the anterior surface of your right finger pads over the posterior surface of your left wrist. Flex your right hand at the metacarpophalangeal joints and place the heel of your right hand over the carpometacarpal joint of your left thumb.

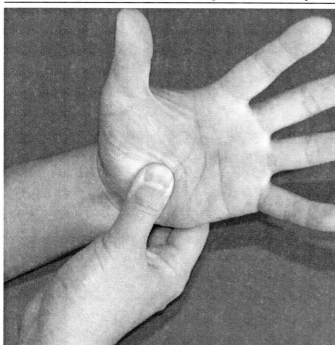

Thumb Pressure over the Carpal Ligaments

2 Place the tip of the right thumb directly over the flexor retinaculum. Do not bend the thumb. Apply heavy pressure while exhaling. Direct this pressure toward the carpal bones and repeat three to five times or as many as desired. Also, adding slight movement in the receiving hand to compensate for the thumb rotation enhances the effectiveness. Reverse the hand position and work the right hand.

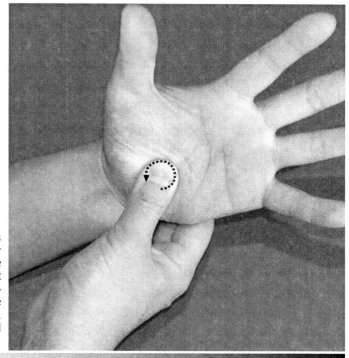

Thumb Rotation on the Carpal Ligaments

3 While applying pressure, as shown in Step 2, add very small rotations. **Rotate the thumb as an entire unit. Do not move from the metacarpophalangeal joint.** Repeat three to five times or as many times as desired. Reverse the hand position and work the right hand.

Kneading the Upper Arm

The purpose of this technique

Reduce tension in the muscles of the upper arm

Area of application

Over the biceps brachii, triceps, and brachioradialis

Description

Examples #1 through #18 demonstrate techniques for hand, wrist, and forearms. The next seven examples help maintain the upper arm, shoulder, and neck. These muscle groups are more developed for working and less problematic than hands and wrists. Should you have time constraints, they may be skipped. As I mentioned in Chapter Two, if maintenance is performed properly, these sets of muscles may require more care.

This example demonstrates kneading over the upper arm, covering the biceps brachii, triceps, and brachioradialis. Tense or aching biceps, triceps, brachioradialis can often inhibit smooth, fluid biomechanics during massage. Too much tension in the elbow and shoulder joints leads to more serious problems later on. Tense biceps and triceps can reduce the flow of energy (*ki*) and blood to the hands, which limits the practitioner's effectiveness. For the massage therapist, the triceps generally need more care than the biceps because of the greater work load they carry.

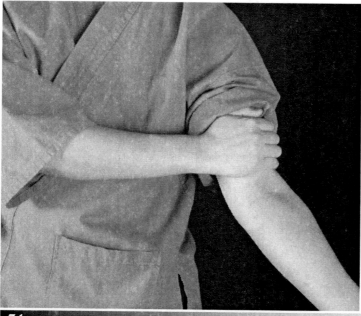

Palm Rotation on the Biceps Brachii

1 Let your left arm hang loosely from your side, with the elbow completely relaxed and the hand resting gently on the massage table. Place the heel of your right hand over the medial edge of your left biceps brachii, just proximal to your elbow. Wrap the fingers of your right hand around the biceps, so that the pads of your four fingers are resting over the lateral edge of the biceps. Keep your thumb out of the way of the working motion.

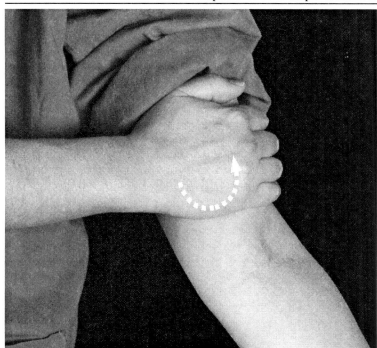

2 Apply firm pressure into the biceps with the heel of your hand and the pads of your fingers, hooking into the underlying tissue. Use the pads of your four fingers as pivots for your hand during the kneading movement. Begin to move your hand in a distal and then lateral direction, gently compressing the tissue into the anterior surface of your four fingers.

3 Release the majority of the pressure, as you move your hand in a proximal and then medial direction to complete the kneading movement. The hand should not break contact with the biceps during the movement slide across the tissue. Complete five to ten rotations or as many as desired. Reposition your hands slightly proximal, repeating the kneading movement. Continue to reposition and repeat the kneading until the entire belly of the muscle has been covered.

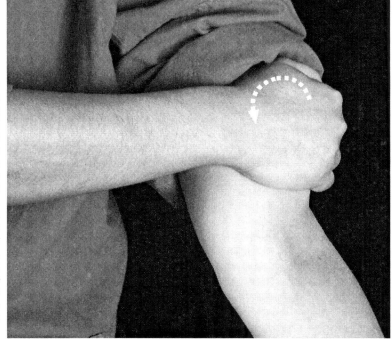

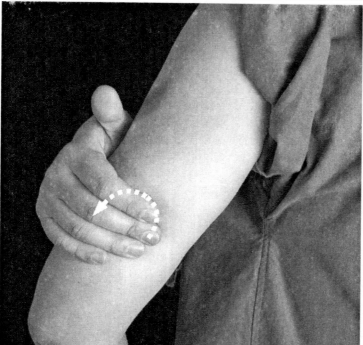

Four-Finger Rotation on the Triceps

4 Rotate your left arm medially from the shoulder joint to bring the triceps into a more accessible position. Place the pads of your four fingers over the medial edge of your left triceps. Wrap your right hand around the triceps with the heel of your hand over the lateral edge of the muscle. For this variation, pivot on the heel of your hand during the kneading movement. Apply firm pressure into the triceps with the heel of your hand and the pads of your fingers, hooking into the underlying tissue. Pull the pads of your fingers in a proximal and then medial direction, gently compressing the tissue against the heel of your hand.

5 Release the majority of the pressure as you move your hand in a distal and then lateral direction to complete the kneading movement. Complete five to ten rotations or as many as desired. Reposition your hands slightly proximal and repeat the kneading movement. Continue to reposition and repeat the kneading until the entire belly of the muscle has been covered. To work the entire muscle, you can rotate the arm slightly to expose different portions of the triceps.

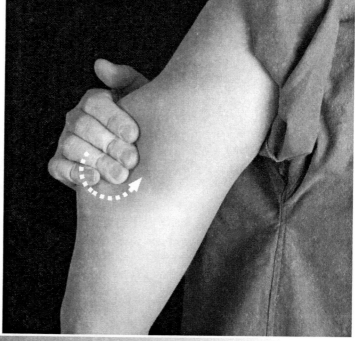

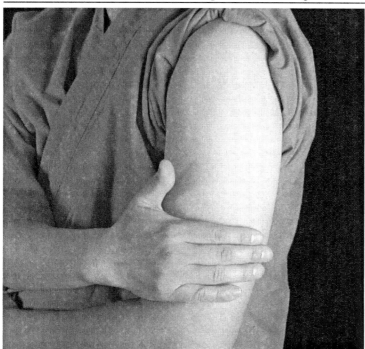

Vibration on the Triceps and Biceps

6 Rotate your left arm medially from the shoulder joint to bring the triceps into a more accessible position. Place the heel of your hand directly over the biceps, just proximal to the elbow. Wrap your right hand around so the fingers reach the triceps. Inhale deeply and, and as you start to exhale, apply a squeezing motion to both the muscles simultaneously and evenly.

7 At the end of the exhalation, begin to vibrate the muscles. Reposition your hands slightly proximal and repeat. Continue to reposition and repeat the squeezing and vibration until the entire belly of the muscle has been covered or until you reach the deltoid. To work the entire muscle, you can rotate the arm slightly to expose different portions of the biceps and triceps. Reverse your hand and body positions and repeat the procedure on your right hand.

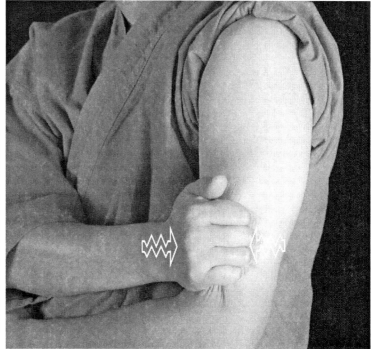

Two-Finger Rotation over the Teres Muscles

The purpose of this technique

Reduce tension in the teres major and minor muscles

Area of application

Over the teres major and minor and the latissimus dorsi

Description

This example demonstrates two-finger rotation over teres major and minor and latissimus dorsi to improve circulation and reduce tension. If anma therapeutic principles are applied properly, teres major and minor will be the used most often, causing them to feel somewhat tight and sore. It is very important that these muscles are kept loose and in optimal condition to maximize therapeutic value. Stimulate the *tsubo* on the scapula (Small Intestine-11, explained in Step 4). It is often very sore, and although sensitive to touch, it is an effective way to loosen tight rotator muscles and relax the entire shoulder region.

Depending upon the person's flexibility or R.O.M., self-massage can have limitations with these muscles. If you need extra care on these regions, another therapist may be able to treat you more effectively than you can treat yourself.

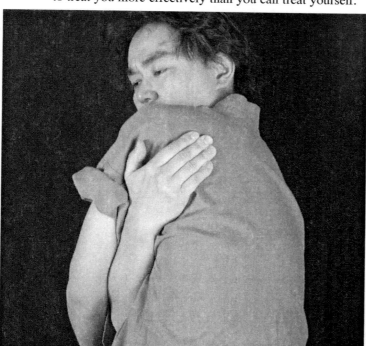

Two-Finger Rotation on Teres Major and Minor

1 Adduct your left arm across your body to protract your left scapula and give you better access to the teres muscles. Place the pads of the middle and ring fingers of your right hand over the teres minor muscle, just medial to the axillary border of the scapula, and inferior to the infraspinatus.

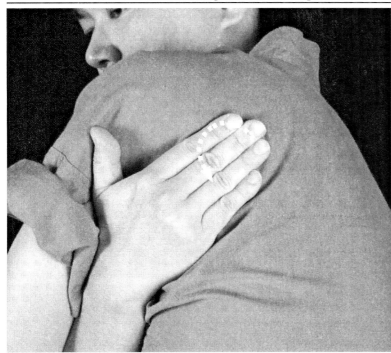

2 Apply firm pressure with the pads of your fingers into the muscle and pull them in a slightly lateral direction, hooking into the underlying tissue. Begin to move the pads of your fingers in a superior and then anterior direction. Continue to move your fingers in an inferior and then posterior direction, returning to the starting position. Complete three to five rotations or as many as desired. Reposition your fingers slightly lateral and repeat the rotation. Continue to slightly reposition your fingers lateral until the entire belly of the muscle has been effectively covered.

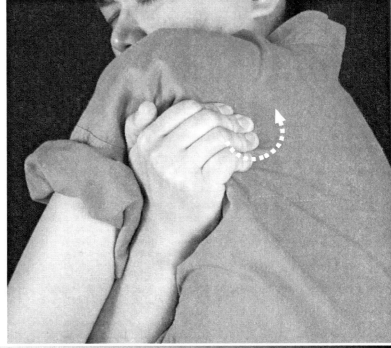

3 Reposition your fingers slightly inferior, directly over the teres major. Repeat the same procedure as described in Step 2 over the teres major. Reverse your hand and body positions and apply the entire procedure to your right side.

Stimulating *Ten So* (Small Intestine-11)

4 Apply pressure or rotation with two fingers on *ten so* (Small Intestine-11). This point can be very sensitive, so adjust the depth and pressure accordingly. Straight pressure is generally used to stimulate this *tsubo*. However, adding small rotations to your movement can disperse the intensity of stimulating this point. This can be a very effective way to treat the rotator muscles while relaxing the entire shoulder region. Apply for five to ten seconds, or as long as desired, and repeat on the other side.

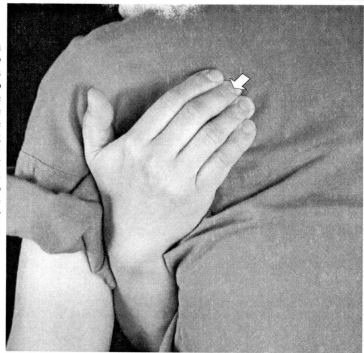

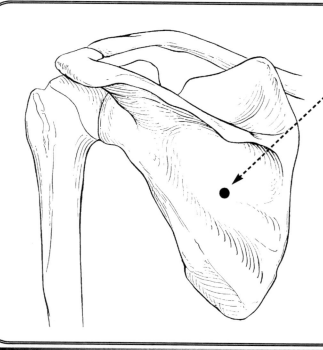

天宗

Ten So—Small Intestine-11

Ten so is located on the horizontal and vertical center of the subscapular fossa, level with the fourth thoracic vertebrae on the infraspinatus muscle.

This point is very effective in treating conditions such as frozen shoulder, numbness on the medial side of the arm and hand, shoulder problems, tennis elbow, whiplash syndrome, and chest pain.

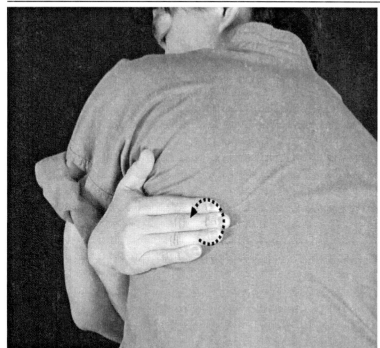

Three-Finger Rotation on the Latissimus Dorsi

5 As you manipulate the teres major and minor muscles, move in an inferior direction and perform rotation on the latissimus dorsi muscle. Adding the index finger to the other fingers makes the working hand more effective. The diameter of the rotation can be slightly larger than that on the teres group. Adjust the amount of pressure according to your sensitivity. Complete five to seven rotations or as many as desired. Reposition your fingers slightly inferior and lateral as needed to perform this technique.

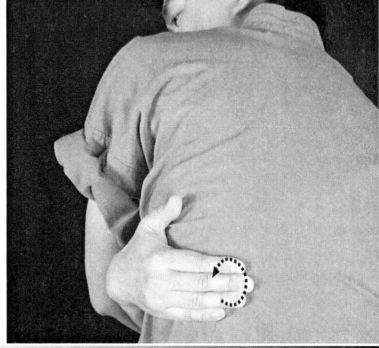

6 Reposition your fingers slightly inferior, directly over the inferior edge of the latissimus dorsi. You can also move in a medial and then lateral direction to cover the entire latissimus dorsi if desired. Repeat the entire procedure over your right side.

Massaging the Deltoid

The purpose of this technique

Reduce muscle tension, prevent injuries, and increase circulation in the deltoid

Area of application

On the deltoid muscles

Description

This example demonstrates three techniques for the deltoid to reduce tension and increase circulation in the muscle. The deltoid carries a large amount of anatomical responsibility due its location and muscular function, and as with the triceps and biceps muscles, tight deltoid muscles can greatly inhibit biomechanical efficiency.

It is very important to maintain this muscle group properly to keep it functioning well and prevent shoulder joint problems. If excessive deltoid tension and limited R.O.M. are being experienced, you should reexamine your body mechanics and make any necessary corrections, ensuring that movements come from the whole body and not just the deltoid/shoulder joint.

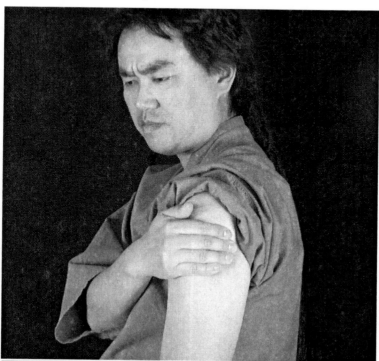

Kneading the Deltoid

1 Let your left arm hang loosely and focus on keeping your shoulder soft and relaxed. Place the heel of your right hand over the anterior fibers of the deltoid and wrap your hand around the muscle, with the pads of your four fingers over the posterior fibers of the deltoid. Your right hand should conform to the contours of your shoulder.

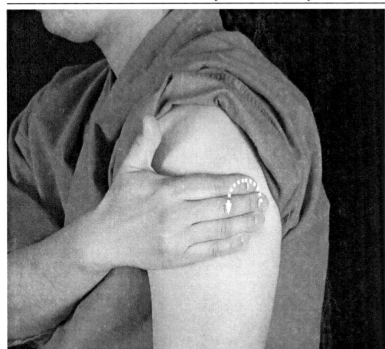

2 Apply pressure with the heel of your hand to compress the anterior deltoid toward the pads of your fingers. Slowly release the pressure with the heel of your hand and apply pressure with the pads of your fingers, pulling them in an anterior direction to compress the posterior deltoid against the palm of your hand.

3 This kneading motion should be smooth and fluid, applying equal pressure to both the anterior and posterior deltoid. Apply the kneading for ten to fifteen seconds or as long as desired. Reverse your hand and body positions and repeat the entire procedure over your right shoulder.

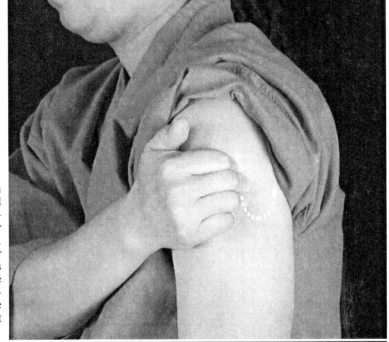

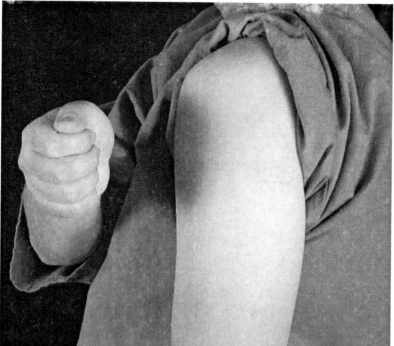

Percussion on the Deltoid

4 Gently bend the right hand and apply percussion to the deltoid. This movement originates from the elbow, with the wrist remaining fairly loose. The palm of the hand should contact the anterior deltoid while the fingers simultaneously contact the posterior deltoid. Move in a slightly proximal and distal direction with each progressing percussion.

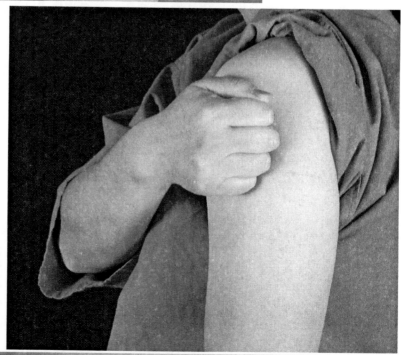

5 Apply the kneading for ten to fifteen seconds or as long as desired. Reverse your hand and body positions and repeat the entire procedure over your right deltoid.

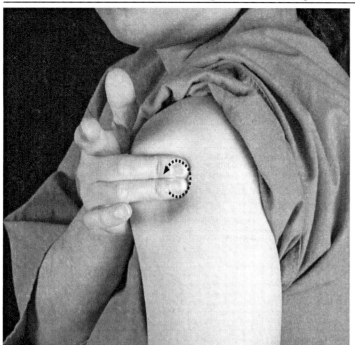

Two-Finger Rotation on
Ken Gu (Large Intestine-15)

6 Apply pressure with the tips of two fingers, using either the index and middle or the ring and middle fingers. Your fingers should slightly overlap while working on *ken gu*. Make very small rotations with the fingertips. This technique helps to loosen shoulder tension and relieve any pain. This *tsubo* is generally very sore on many therapists; therefore, adjust the amount of pressure according to your sensitivity level. Knead for ten to fifteen seconds or as long as desired. Reverse your hand and body positions and repeat the entire procedure over your right deltoid.

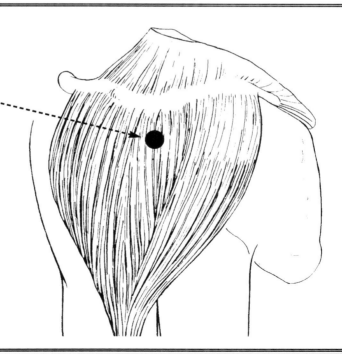

肩髃

**Ken Gu—
Large Intestine-15**

Ken gu is located just distal and anterior to the acromian in the anterior depression of the deltoid muscle at the attachment of the supraspinatus. Should you have difficulty locating this point, palpate the area until you find a spot that seems to be particularly sensitive and apply this technique there.

Palm Rotation over the Pectoralis Muscles

The purpose of this technique

Reduce tension and increase circulation in the pectoralis muscles

Area of application

Over the pectoralis major and minor muscles

Description

This example demonstrates palm rotation over the pectoralis major and minor to reduce tension and increase circulation to the muscles. Pectoralis minor is used quite often during massage therapy and tends to become tense and very sensitive. Gentle palm rotation is usually sufficient; however, if you need deeper stimulation and can tolerate the deeper work, you can try using the tips of two or three fingers on the pectoralis minor muscle.

After the pectoralis major begins to loosen with self-care, you will feel a tough fiber, the pectoralis minor, superficial to the pectoralis major. This muscle runs diagonally from the shoulder. Due to its generally tight nature, this muscle can greatly inhibit breathing, flexibility, and overall body efficiency. I highly recommend that you keep this muscle in proper working order to maintain good health.

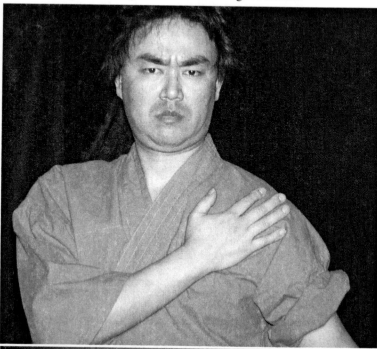

1 Place the heel of your right hand over your left pectoralis major, just medial to your left anterior deltoid. Your fingers and thumb should conform to the contours of your chest and shoulder.

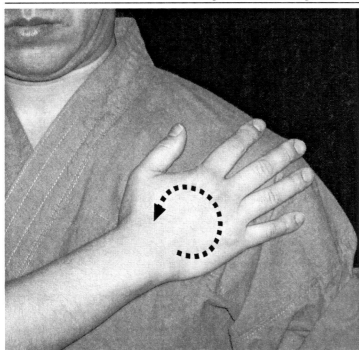

2 Apply firm pressure with the heel of your right hand, hooking into the underlying tissue. Use the pads of your fingers as pivots for your hand during the rotation. Begin to move the heel of your hand in a proximal and then lateral direction. Continue to move your hand in a distal and then medial direction, returning to the starting position. Complete five to ten rotations or as many as desired.

3 Reposition your hand slightly medial and repeat Step 2. Continue to reposition your hand medially and repeat the procedure until the entire muscle has been covered. Female therapists can use the left hand to move the breast tissue in different directions, allowing greater access to the underlying muscle. **To prevent tissue damage, do not apply this technique over or through the breast tissue.** Reverse your hand and body positions and repeat Steps 1 through 3 over your right pectoralis major with your left hand.

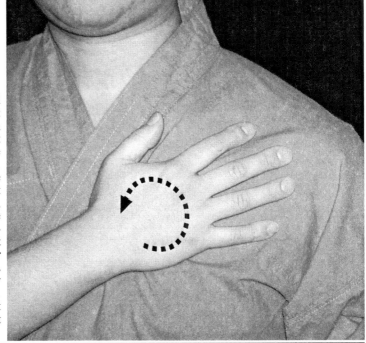

Rotation on the Upper Trapezius

The purpose of this technique

Reduce tension in the upper trapezius and shoulders

Area of application

Over the upper trapezius between the shoulders and the neck

Description

This example demonstrates several techniques for reducing tension in the upper back muscles such as the trapezius, levator scapulae, rhomboid minor, supraspinatus, and infraspinatus. Upper back tension and backache are not just uncomfortable but restrict the movement of the scapula and shoulder. Some scapulae have adhered to the underlying tissue, which restricts the movement of the rotator cuffs and limits the range of motion of the arms. It also restricts blood (*ki*) flow to the arms and hands. Therefore, proper loosening of the upper back and shoulder is essential to maintain quality of treatment.

Although daily self-massage of the upper back can be of great personal benefit, there are limitations due to the natural R.O.M. Receiving frequent bodywork to maintain optimum conditioning is suggested.

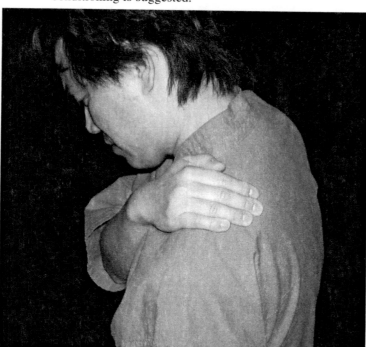

Three-Finger Rotation on the Suprascapular Region

1 Stand or sit in a relaxed position with your left arm hanging loosely. Place the flat, anterior surface of your right index, middle, and ring fingers over the upper trapezius, just medial to the acromion process.

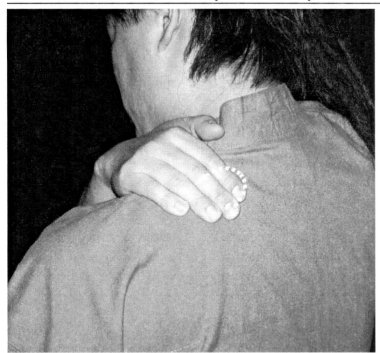

2 Apply firm pressure with the flat, anterior surface of your right index, middle, and ring fingers into the upper trapezius, hooking into the muscle. Begin to move your hand medially and anteriorly, gliding over the underlying tissue, but not sliding over the skin or clothing.

3 Continue to move your hand in a lateral and then posterior direction, returning to the starting position. Complete five to seven rotations or as many as desired. Continue to reposition your hand slightly medial and repeat the rotation until the entire suprascapular region has been effectively covered.

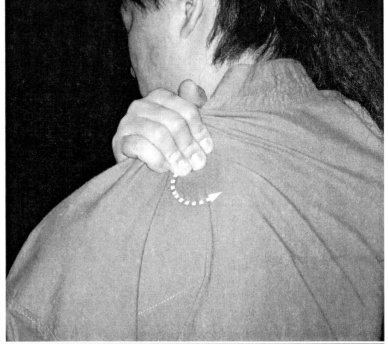

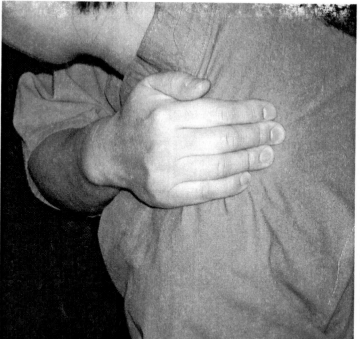

Squeeze and Vibrate the Suprascapular Region

4 Place the flat, anterior surface of your right four fingers directly over your left upper trapezius, with the tips of the fingers touching the proximal edge of the spine of the scapula. The heel of your hand should rest directly on your left clavicle. Apply firm pressure with the pads of your fingers, hooking into the underlying tissue. Pull your fingers anterior, compressing the tissue into the heel of your hand. Your fingers should flex at the metacarpophalangeal and proximal interphalangeal joints, and the distal interphalangeal joints should slightly hyperextend. **Do not apply pressure with your fingertips.**

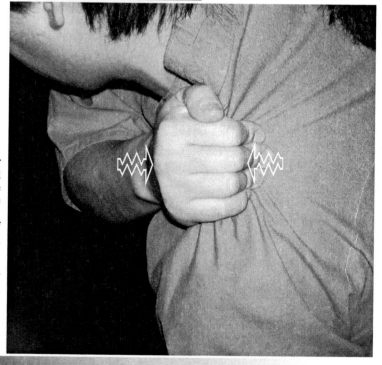

5 Hold the compression for three to five seconds and release. You may add fine vibrations while you are compressing the tissue. Repeat the application of compression and vibration two to three times or as many times as desired. Depending on the size of your body, you may need to slightly reposition your hand and repeat the procedure to cover the entire muscle in the suprascapular region.

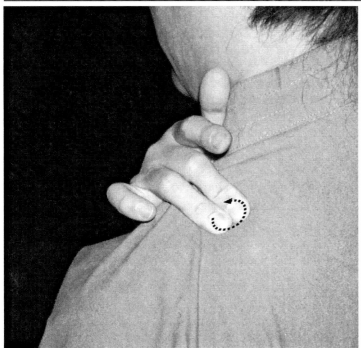

Two-Finger Rotation on Supraspinatus

6 Apply pressure toward the scapula by inserting the tips of two fingers, either index and middle or ring and middle fingers. Hook the fingers into the supraspinatus and pull the working hand toward your front (anterior) side. When working on the supraspinatus, make very small rotations with the fingertips in the medial, proximal, lateral, and distal directions. As you rotate, move medially to laterally to cover the entire muscle. This technique loosens shoulder tension and relieves any pain that may be present. Apply the kneading for ten to fifteen seconds or as long as desired. Reverse your hand and body positions and repeat the entire procedure over your right supraspinatus.

Two-Finger Rotation on Infraspinatus

7 Continue the procedure as in Step 6 but move the hand inferior to reach and cover the infraspinatus. This technique is dependent on your personal flexibility. Should your R.O.M. not allow you to reach this far, then omit the procedure. Complete five to seven rotations or as many as desired. Reposition your hand slightly medial or lateral until the entire infraspinatus has been effectively covered. Apply the kneading for ten to fifteen seconds or as long as desired. Reverse your hand and body positions and repeat the entire procedure over your right infraspinatus.

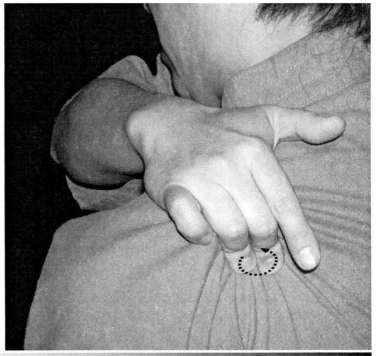

Kneading the Neck

The purpose of this technique

Reduce tension and increase circulation and flexibility in the neck

Area of application

Over the muscles of the posterior neck

Description

Reducing neck tension is very important for the flexibility of the entire back. For example, if the cervical attachment of the trapezius is tense, the shoulder attachment will be as well. Therefore, to effectively reduce tension of the rotator cuff, you must also reduce the tension in the cervical region. When the muscles of the neck are tight, the upper thoracic area and the scapula compensate, leaving the entire upper back tense. To loosen the upper back, it is very important that the neck is also loose. This example demonstrates massaging the muscles of the posterior neck to reduce tension and increase circulation to the area.

This technique can be easier to apply when lying in the supine position, because the neck muscles are not supporting the head. Sometimes neck tension can originate in the intrascapular region, and often neck muscles will not loosen until the cervical region has loosened. Should this be the case, it is recommended to seek the aid of another therapist.

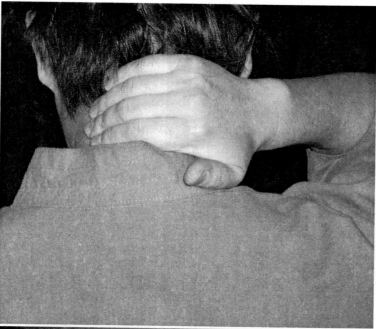

1 This example uses the same kneading movement as previously described in Step 2 and 3 of Example #21, except it is applied over the muscles of the posterior neck. Place the heel of your right hand over the lateral edge of the erector muscles on the right side of your neck. Wrap your hand around the posterior portion of your neck, with the pads of your fingers resting over the lateral edge of the erector muscles on the left side of your neck. Your hand should be soft enough to conform to the contours of your neck.

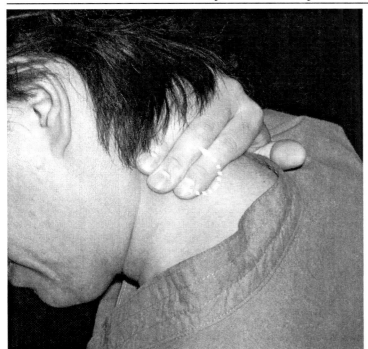

Kneading the Neck

2 Apply pressure with the heel of your hand to compress the erector muscles on the right side toward the spineous processes. Slowly release the pressure with the heel of your hand and apply pressure with the pads of your fingers. Pull in a medial direction to compress the erector muscles on the left side toward the spineous processes.

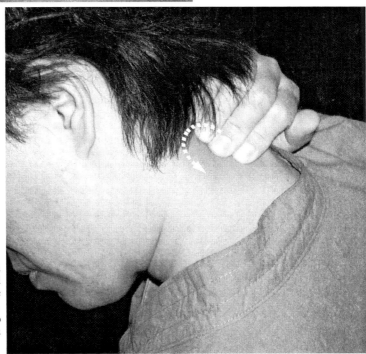

3 This kneading motion should be smooth and fluid, applying equal pressure to both sides of the neck. Apply the kneading for ten to fifteen seconds or as long as desired.

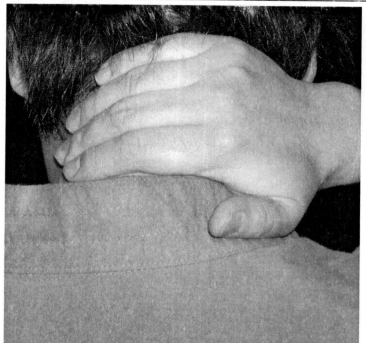

Squeezing the Neck

4 Use the same hand position as described in Step 1. Inhale slowly and deeply, applying firm, equal, pressure with the pads of your four fingers and the heel of your right hand into the erector muscles, to compress them against the spineous processes during exhalation.

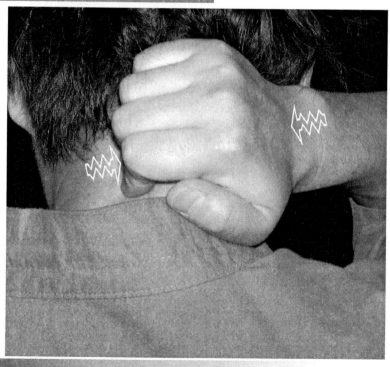

5 Hold the compression for five to seven seconds or as long as desired. Repeat the application of pressure two to three times. **Do not add vibrations to this technique because of the close proximity to the head.**

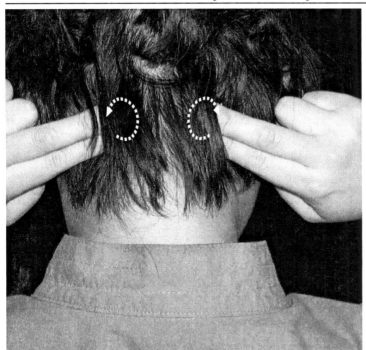

Rotation on the Base of the Skull

6 Place the pads of your index and middle fingers of both hands just inferior to the base of the skull. The starting placement for each hand should be lateral to the spine. Apply light pressure with both hands into the suboccipital region. The left hand stabilizes the skull, while the right hand applies the rotation. Begin to rotate the pads of your fingers from your right hand in small circles over the suboccipital region. Complete three to five rotations or as many as desired.

7 Reposition the fingers of your right hand slightly lateral and repeat the rotation. Continue to reposition your fingers, repeating the procedure until the entire right side of the suboccipital region has been sufficiently covered. **Do not over-stimulate the region or you may cause a headache.** Apply the rotation over the left side of the suboccipital region with your left hand, while your right hand stabilizes the skull.

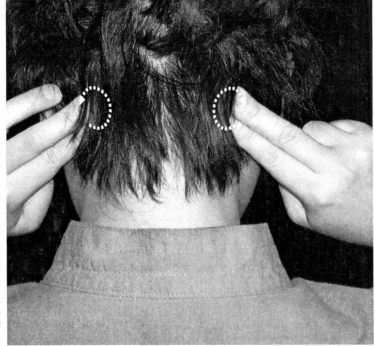

Stretching the Shoulders Three Ways

The purpose of this technique

Stretch the deltoid, pectoralis, triceps, latissimus dorsi, and teres major and minor muscles

Area of application

Around the shoulders

Description

These three stretching techniques for the shoulders, back, and chest loosen the upper back and shoulders. These stretches work best when applied in conjunction with exhalation. I highly recommend the practice of some type of physical exercise, such as Tai Chi or Yoga, to be used in conjunction with body work, as it greatly increases the fluidity of body movement, increases energy (*ki*), and generally raises the level of life force. This increased vitality is of great benefit to the practice of body therapy.

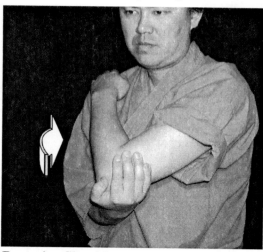 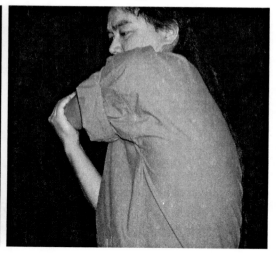

Posterior Shoulder

1 Stand with your feet apart, slightly wider than shoulder-width. Gently cup your left elbow with your right hand and adduct your left arm across your body. Inhale slowly and deeply and as you exhale, gently pull your left elbow across your body. Pull your arm to the limit of your R.O.M. and then slightly past this point to gently stretch the posterior deltoid, infraspinatus, and rhomboid muscles. You may rotate your torso in the same direction to enhance the stretch.

2 Release the stretch at the end of your exhalation. **Do not overstretch the muscles.** Repeat the stretch two to three times or as many times as desired. **Always apply the stretch while you exhale.** Reverse your hand and body positions and repeat the stretch on your right side.

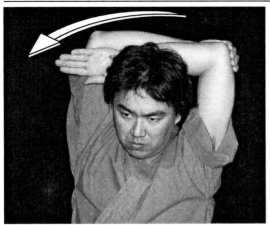

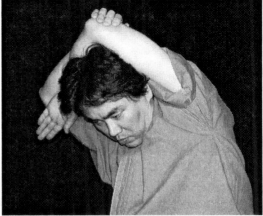

Latissimus Dorsi and Teres Major and Minor

3 Flex and abduct the shoulder of your right arm and then flex your elbow, so the forearm and hand are posterior to your head. Cup your left elbow with your right hand. Inhale slowly and deeply and as you exhale, gently pull your right elbow behind your head to abduct the arm and laterally flex your torso.

4 Pull your arm to the limit of your range of motion and then slightly past this point to gently stretch the latissimus dorsi, and teres major and minor muscles. Release the stretch at the end of your exhalation. Repeat the stretch two to three times or as many times as desired. Reverse your hand and body positions and repeat the stretch on your left side.

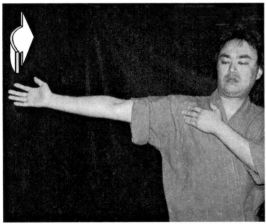

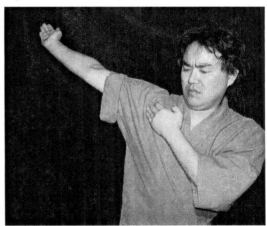

Pectoralis Major

5 Stand with your feet apart, slightly wider than shoulder-width. Place the pads of the four fingers of your left hand over the fibers of your right anterior deltoid. Abduct your right shoulder, so the upper arm is relatively horizontal. Inhale slowly and deeply and as you exhale, rotate your torso to your right side to the limit of your R.O.M.

6 Then, apply pressure with your left hand into your anterior deltoid to push the shoulder slightly past the limit of your R.O.M. to gently stretch your pectoralis major. Release the stretch at the end of your exhalation. Repeat the stretch two to three times or as many times as desired. Reverse your hand and body positions and repeat the stretch on your left side.

Chapter Four

Ancient Wisdom

When a culture can measure its history in millennia rather than in centuries, there are sure to be very strong traditions which underlie the stability of the culture and act as binding forces to keep the minds and hearts of the people together. When traditions produce excellence over countless generations, a great deal of confidence develops in the people who are part of that culture. This is because the traditions continually benefit the culture. When something is seen to bring harm to a culture, it is identified and rejected. Obviously, when a culture has survived and flourished for thousands of years, it arrives at many points of wisdom which it would not sacrifice at any cost. There are traditional principles for ruling, farming, healing, raising families, and resolving disputes. Although these traditions constantly undergo examination and evolution, the underlying principles rarely change. When a set of underlying principles is kept intact despite the evolution of a tradition, it is because they have been recognized to contain wisdom. Ancient traditions preserve essential principles which enable a culture to evolve along pathways that are marked and shepherded by principles of wisdom.

Therefore, when we study an ancient tradition, we are exposed to something extremely rich, which unfolds itself in a way that is fine-tuned to the experience of learning by a progressive method. It is a delight to come into the realm of traditional training, because we are certain to succeed in our study and training if we follow the course through which countless students like ourselves have succeeded in the past. In the path that these students and masters have passed on to us, we discover something very precious: there is wisdom in the tradition, and the tradition brings about definite results. We realize that by following the encouragement and advice that has been so generously laid out for us, we do in fact achieve excellence, and we become the holders of that traditional knowledge.

When I asked my master, "How can I find the essential points within the variety of teachings?" he responded, "When we seek the truth, we must observe that which comes and goes and that which remains." This was quite a profound response. He meant that there are always elements within a tradition that are not crucial but have become suddenly popular and are presently flourishing, even though they do not last. Every tradition has such examples. There are always masters who introduce something to a tradition, built from fundamental principles and serving a need for a time before vanishing from the tradition completely. We know of many such stories in Japanese massage. What is important for the student is to recognize what fundamental principles of the tradition that are indisputably necessary and will never vanish. Within the tradition of massage therapy, it is certain that hand maintenance and body mechanics are elements of the tradition which are essential. These teachings are not temporary fads—without them massage would not have been able to develop as it has. Practitioners of the past millennia would have given up massage because of physical injury, and they would not have been able to pass this knowledge on to us! We can confidently identify hand maintenance and body mechanics as essential components to the vitality and continuity of the art itself.

There is great respect for the traditional arts in Japan because it is known that a practitioner must go through deep training to gain the experience and skill necessary to deliver a competent performance. When one is finally able to give such a performance, it is certain to be of a profound and moving nature—the training guarantees it. Without this training, the performance is not authentic. It may appear similar but is obviously not the genuine thing; it is devoid of real substance, and an intelligent observer can see this. Any traditional art takes significant time to master and when this time is invested, one learns the art in a genuine way. It is only a matter of dedication.

In the United States, a full-time massage therapist gives about twenty-five massage sessions a week. In Japan, the standard load for a full-time massage therapist in a week is forty-five to fifty sessions. Despite this great number of massages, forearm, hand, and wrist problems are extremely rare in Japan. Why is this? Because Japanese massage therapists are trained in a traditional procedure of hand maintenance, with an emphasis on recognizing and avoiding specific movements that can deteriorate the health and functioning of the hands.

As an example of the effectiveness of these techniques, I can offer you my own experience, which is typical of professional training in Japan. I have been performing massage since my youth and have gone through the traditional training methods. The muscles in my hands have developed through years of application in conjunction with hand maintenance routines. Now they are strong and healthy enough to require little maintenance, even with a full schedule of massage sessions. This is the result of years of attention to the basics. If new therapists want to attain a professional's level of hand strength and health, they should do so by applying the traditional methods of hand maintenance, which relieve stress and pain and help the muscles to develop optimum strength and health. The routine of hand maintenance techniques presented in this book contains the essential practices that have kept Japanese massage therapists healthy through vigorous massage schedules over the years. I encourage you to learn these techniques and incorporate them into your daily massage practice. As an old Japanese proverb says, "An ounce of prevention is worth a pound of cure."

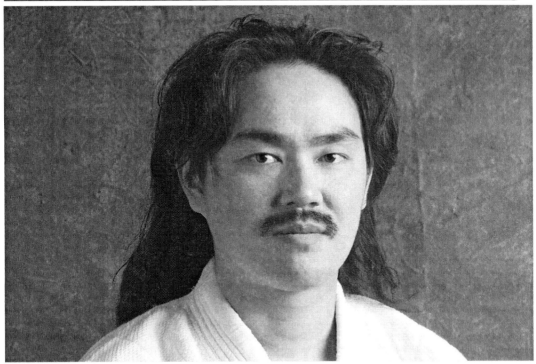

I have tried very hard to describe traditional techniques accurately but there are limitations to studying massage from a book, regardless of the number of photographs and illustrations. Massage is a subtle art beyond the reach of words. Since it is not possible for me to be with all students interested in learning traditions of Japanese massage, this book can serve as a reference during the preliminary stage of study. If you are interested in further training, have any questions, comments or suggestions about the material covered in this book, or if you want information about my workshops, feel free to contact me. Thanks again to all those people who show interest in our way of healing.

Good health to you!

Shogo Mochizuki

c/o Kotobuki Publications
P.O. Box 19917
Boulder, CO   80308-2917
www.japanesemassge.org

HAND MAINTENANCE TECHNIQUES
QUICK REFERENCES

Example #1. Palm Rotation over the Forearms

Example #2. Two-Finger Rotation on the Brachioradialis Muscle

Example #3. Kneading the Brachioradialis

Example #4. Percussion on the Forearms

Example #5. Thumb Pressure on the Radius and Ulna

Example #6. Two-Finger Rotation on the Posterior Forearm

Example #7. Rotation over the Wrist

Example #8. Fascial Release on the Wrist

Example #9. Deep Rotation on the Muscles of the Palm

Example #10. Stroking between the Metacarpals with the Thumbs

Example #11. Massage around *Go Koku*

Example #12. Light Stroking on the Fingers

Example #13. Thumb Rotation on the Joints of the Fingers

Example #14. Traction and Decompression of the Fingers

Example #15. Interlocking and Stretching the Fingers

Example #16. Gentle Stretching of the Wrist

Example #17. Stretching between the Metacarpals by Compressing the Palm

Example #18. Pressure and Rotation on the Carpal Ligaments

Example #19. Kneading the Upper Arm

Example #20. Two-Finger Rotation over the Teres Muscles

Example #21. Massaging the Deltoid

Example #22. Palm Rotation over the Pectoralis Muscles

Example #23. Rotation on the Upper Trapezius

Example #24. Kneading the Neck

Example #25. Stretching the Shoulders Three Ways

© Kotobuki Publications

Related Materials
Available from
Kotobuki Publications

Kotobuki Popular Editions

The popular editions have been extracted from the professional editions of our publications. We have selected easy-to-learn techniques that give step-by-step instructions for laypeople, massage therapists, students, and various health professionals. We have also minimized the professional anatomical and medical terminology so anyone can enjoy and benefit from the popular editions. Videos are available to supplement the textbooks as visual aids, and they demonstrate all examples in the textbooks. However, the videos do not contain basic, important information, such as the precautions, set-up procedures, and concepts. The videos are created specifically to act as a visual supplementation for use with the textbooks, and therefore are not sold independently (call for information).

Ko Bi Do™ : The Art of Japanese Facial Massage
Popular Edition

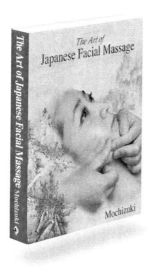

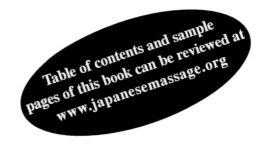

Table of contents and sample pages of this book can be reviewed at www.japanesemassage.org

This book features:

- Application techniques of Japanese facial massage
- Japanese concepts of health and beauty
- 45 examples for the face and neck
- Over 300 detailed photos and illustrations
- 187 pgs softcover, ISBN 1-57615-053-4

Book only $ 19.⁹⁵

Ko bi do: Japanese facial massage is different from every other method of facial massage. It uniquely combines the very effective methods of facial massage with traditional East Asian concepts. Forty-five examples of techniques covering the face and neck are demonstrated throughout the three different stages of application. Over 300 photographs and illustrations supplement over 187 pages of detailed text.

Ko bi do™: Ancient Way of Beauty
The Art of Japanese Facial Massage
Book & Video Set

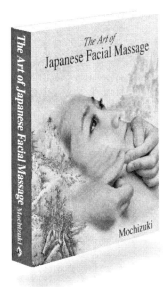
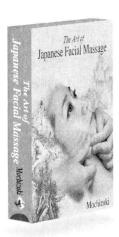

This video supplements the popular edition of *The Art of Japanese Facial Massage* with vivid demonstrations of each of the forty-five easy-to-learn examples found in the textbook. It also demonstrates how to combine the techniques to construct a full-facial massage. All demonstrations are done by Shogo Mochizuki.

This video features:

- Basic facial massage application techniques
- 45 application examples for the face and neck
- Demonstration of three-stage facial massage treatment
- Approx. 60 minutes running time.
- ISBN 1-57615-054-2

Book and Video set $ 59.⁹⁰   ISBN 1-57615-055-0

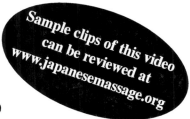
Sample clips of this video can be reviewed at www.japanesemassage.org

ANMA
The Art of Japanese Massage
Popular Edition

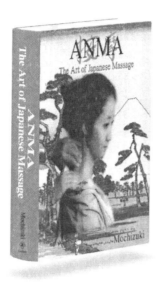

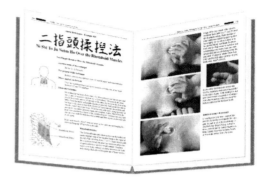

We selected **forty-five examples** of easy-to-learn techniques with step-by-step instructions. Complemented with over **300 photographs and illustrations**, this text comprehensively explains the art and methods of anma.

Anma originated in China over 4,000 years ago and was introduced to Japan about 1,300 years ago. Swedish massage and shiatsu are among the massage forms which grew out of this rich tradition. This book is the popular edition of *Anma: The Art of Japanese Massage*. It is the first Japanese-authored massage book published in English about anma.

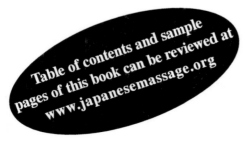

Table of contents and sample pages of this book can be reviewed at www.japanesemassage.org

This book features:

- History and principles of anma
- Anma application techniques
- 45 application examples for the entire body
- Over 300 detailed photos and illustrations
- 199 pgs softcover,   ISBN 1-57615-050-X

Book only $ 19.⁹⁵

ANMA
Book & Video Set

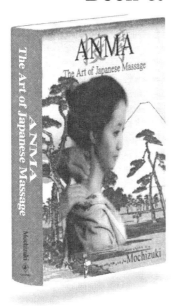

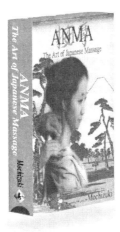

This video supplements the popular edition of *Anma: The Art of Japanese Massage*. It demonstrates forty-five easy-to-learn examples and visually supplements the textbook. It also demonstrates how to combine the techniques to construct a smooth, therapeutic full-body massage. Demonstrated by Shogo Mochizuki.

This video features:

- Nine categories of anma application techniques
- 45 application examples for the entire body
- Approx. 60 minutes running time
- ISBN 1-57615-051-8

**Book and Video set $ 59.^{90} ISBN 1-57615-052-6

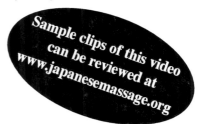

Sample clips of this video can be reviewed at www.japanesemassage.org

Zoku Shin Do™
The Art of Japanese Foot Massage
Popular Edition

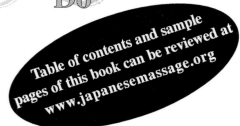

Table of contents and sample pages of this book can be reviewed at www.japanesemassage.org

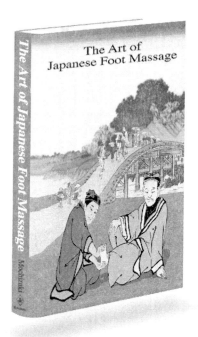

This book features:

- Application techniques of Japanese foot massage
- Brief history and principles of zoku shin do
- 45 examples of applications for the foot
- Over 300 detailed photos and illustrations
- 191 pgs softcover,   ISBN 1-57615-056-9

Book Only $ 19.⁹⁵

Zoku shin do, the oldest known form of East Asian foot reflexology, originated in China over five thousand years ago. **The Art of Japanese Foot Massage** explains the method of foot massage that arose from this ancient tradition. Forty-five easy-to-follow examples of foot-massage techniques are shown. This book also includes detailed explanations of meridians, and pressure points. Over 300 photographs and illustrations span this 191 page volume.

Zoku Shin Do™
The Art of Japanese Foot Massage
Book & Video Set

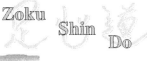

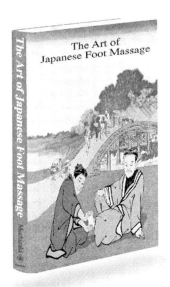

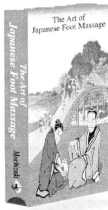

This video supplements the text of *The Art of Japanese Foot Massage*. It demonstrates all forty-five easy-to-learn examples found in the textbook. It also demonstrates how to combine these techniques seamlessly to construct a therapeutic foot massage. Demonstrated by Shogo Mochizuki.

This video features:

- Basic foot application techniques
- 45 application examples for the foot
- Demonstrates how to combine techniques
- Approx. 60 minutes running time
- ISBN 1-57615-057-7

Book and Video set $ 59.⁹⁰   ISBN 1-57615-058-5

Kotobuki Professional Editions

The professional editions are written for massage therapists and students. They use common medical terminology, such as the names of muscles and bones. These books are intended for professionals and students who already have basic massage training.

Hand Maintenance Guide
for Massage Therapists
Professional Edition

Understanding how to maintain your hands and prevent injuries is very important for massage therapists. This book will explain thirteen of the most common contraindicated movements in massage therapy which have been proven to cause hand and wrist problems along with providing solutions to avoid injury. This book also explains twenty-five common massage techniques that will help you optimize the condition of your arms and hands. This knowledge has been derived from 1,300 years of massage education in Japan. **This is absolutely a MUST HAVE for the massage practitioner!**

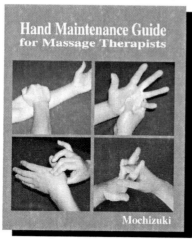

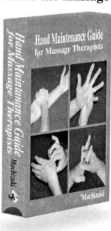

This Book Features:

- Why hand maintenance is necessary
- Cause of problems
- 25 examples of hand maintenance techniques
- Over 170 detailed photos and illustrations
- 101 pgs softcover, ISBN 1-57615-075-5

Book Only $ 19.⁹⁵

This video features:

- Cause of problems
- 25 examples of hand main. techniques
- Approx. 40 minutes running time
- ISBN 1-57615-076-3

Book and Video set **$ 59.⁹⁰** ISBN 1-57615-077-1

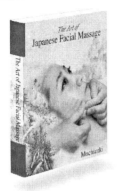
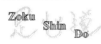
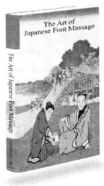

Japanese Chair-Massage Techniques
Professional Edition

Chair massage is the fastest-growing adjunct modality for massage therapists. Anma (traditional Japanese massage) and shiatsu are non-oil massage techniques that will change and enhance your way of giving a chair massage, maximizing the therapeutic value. Mochizuki, one of the most knowledgeable and experienced instructors in North America, draws upon over 240 years of family expertise to demonstrate how the Japanese massage techniques work with the massage chair. Each of these comprehensive textbooks offers 55 easy-to-follow, detailed examples supplemented by over 300 photographs and illustrations. Volume One explains all the basics of Japanese massage and demonstrates the techniques for the back, shoulders, neck, and hips from the back position. Volume Two demonstrates additional techniques for the shoulders, arms, and hands from the front position. Traditional Japanese hand reflexology is also explained.

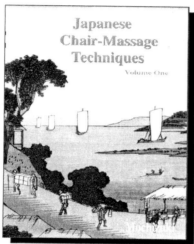

Volume Two Features:

- 55 techniques applied from the front
- 25 techniques applied from the Side
- 5 techniques for a finishing touch
- Over 600 detailed photos and illustrations
- 289 pgs softcover,   ISBN 1-57615-081-X

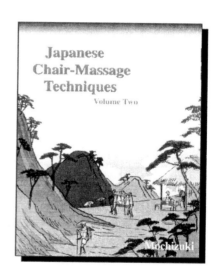

Volume One Features:

- Application techniques of Japanese chair massage
- Principles of Japanese massage
- 55 examples of techniques applied from the back
- Over 300 detailed photos and illustrations
- 229 pgs Softcover,   ISBN 1-57615-078-X

Textbooks only

•Volume One: $40.^{00} ISBN 1-57615-078-X
•Volume Two: $40.^{00} ISBN 1-57615-081-X

Textbooks and instructional videos

•Volume One: textbook and video set: $199.^{95} ISBN 1-57615-080-1
•Volume Two: textbook and video set: $199.^{95} ISBN 1-57615-083-6

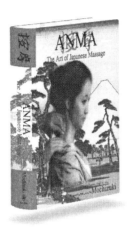
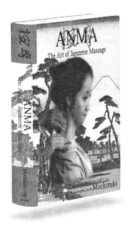
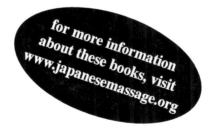

Japanese Massage
Intensive Workshops

The Japanese Massage and Bodywork Institute in Boulder, Colorado offers intensive workshops several times each year. Smaller seminars are also available throughout the United States, Europe and Brazil. For information and the dates of these programs, call us or visit our website.

ANMA: The Art of Japanese Massage
Certification Course

Ninety percent of this course will involve hands-on training, but there will also be an introduction to North East Asian medical theory including tsubo, meridian theory and diagnosis. Our classes combine *koho* anma (traditional anma) and *genko* anma (modern anma). *Koho* anma is the therapeutic core of anma practice. This is a rare opportunity to study directly with one of the most experienced and knowledgeable anma instructors/practitioners.

Japanese Chair-Massage Techniques
Certification Course

Chair Massage is the fastest growing adjunct modality for massage therapists. After seven years of development, drawing from an extensive repertoire of both anma and shiatsu, Mochizuki has developed this modality to bring chair massage to its highest therapeutic potential. Ninety percent of this course will involve hands-on training. These arts are best suited for chair massage for they are non-oil based and applied over clothing, which is typical to chair massage. This course will be supported by and draw upon the most thorough textbooks within the art.

The Art of Japanese Facial Massage
Certification Course

Japanese Facial Massage is different from every other method of facial massage. It uniquely combines modern methods of facial massage with traditional East Asian concepts. Japanese facial massage techniques originated in anma, and were further refined in the field of cosmetology to effectively work on the face. They are performed very lightly with smooth stroking and quick, light, percussive techniques. The stimulation is not heavy, but it affects the underlying tissues to increase the blood circulation, enhance the condition of the skin and minimize the aging process.

In this course you will learn:
- Three stages of facial massage treatment: cleansing, moisturizing, and energizing
- Basic and advanced facial technique
- Neck and shoulder massage
- Descriptions and locations of *keiraku* (meridians) and tsubo (acupoints) on the face
- Facelift techniques using tsubo (acupoints) and meridians
- Masque and exfoliation
- Product selection for various skin types
- Basic Japanese foot massage

Zoku Shin Do Reflexology
Certification Course

Zoku shin do (traditional East Asian foot reflexology), is the oldest known form of reflexology, originating in China over five thousand years ago. Zoku shin do uniquely combines foot massage, *keiraku* (meridian concepts), tsubo (acupoints), *Zo Fu Hansha* (internal organ reflection), and *Keiraku Hansha* (meridian reflection theory) to balance the physical and psychological aspects of the client. It is based on the Yin/Yang, Five Elements, and Meridian theorem, rather than the Zone theory of Western Reflexology. The foot is the foundation of the body's structure and health. Japanese foot massage combines very fast, light, and smooth techniques along with slow, deep, stimulating techniques to enhance the client's health. It was originally developed by zoku shin do practitioners as a warm-up exercise for both the client and the practitioner. Reflexology is not considered massage therapy, therefore, there are no prerequisites for this class.